The Ideal of Nature

The Ideal of Nature

Debates about Biotechnology and the Environment

Edited by

Gregory E. Kaebnick

Scholar and Editor, *Hastings Center Report*
The Hastings Center
Garrison, New York

The Johns Hopkins University Press
Baltimore

The Johns Hopkins University Press
2715 North Charles Street
Baltimore, Maryland 21218-4363
www.press.jhu.edu

Library of Congress Cataloging-in-Publication Data
The ideal of nature : debates about biotechnology and the environment /
edited by Gregory E. Kaebnick.
        p. ; cm.
   Includes bibliographical references and index.
   ISBN-13: 978-0-8018-9888-4 (hardcover : alk. paper)
   ISBN-10: 0-8018-9888-9 (hardcover : alk. paper)
1. Bioethics. 2. Biotechnology—Moral and ethical aspects.
3. Nature—Effect of human beings on. I. Kaebnick, Gregory E.
   [DNLM: 1. Biotechnology—ethics—United States—Essays.
2. Genetic Engineering—ethics—United States—Essays. 3. Agricul-
ture—United States—Essays. 4. Bioethical Issues—United States—
Essays. 5. Nature—United States—Essays. 6. Public Policy—United
States—Essays. WB 60]
   QH332.I337 2011
   179'.1—dc22   2010042481

A catalog record for this book is available from the British Library.

*Special discounts are available for bulk purchases of this book. For
more information, please contact Special Sales at 410-516-6936 or
specialsales@press.jhu.edu.*

The Johns Hopkins University Press uses environmentally friendly book
materials, including recycled text paper that is composed of at least
30 percent post-consumer waste, whenever possible.

Contents

Contributors

Nicholas Agar, Ph.D., Associate Professor and Head, Philosophy Programme, Victoria University of Wellington, Wellington, New Zealand

William Galston, Ph.D., Ezra Zilkha Chair, Governance Studies, The Brookings Institution, Washington, D.C.

Bruce Jennings, M.A., Director of Bioethics, Center for Humans and Nature, New York, New York

Gregory E. Kaebnick, Ph.D., Scholar and editor of the *Hastings Center Report,* The Hastings Center, Garrison, New York

Eric Katz, Ph.D., Professor of Philosophy, Department of Humanities, Science, Technology, and Society Program, New Jersey Institute of Technology, Newark, New Jersey

Paul Lauritzen, M.A., Ph.D., Director, Program in Applied Ethics, Department of Religious Studies, John Carroll University, University Heights, Ohio

Peter Murray, doctoral candidate, University at Albany–SUNY, Albany, New York

Thomas H. Murray, Ph.D., President, The Hastings Center, Garrison, New York

Jean Porter, Ph.D., John A. O'Brien Professor of Theological Ethics, Department of Theology, Notre Dame University, Notre Dame, Indiana

Kate Soper, M.A., Professor Emerita, Institute for the Study of European Transformations, London Metropolitan University, London, United Kingdom

Bonnie Steinbock, Ph.D., Professor, Department of Philosophy, University at Albany–SUNY, Albany, New York

Steven Vogel, Ph.D., Brickman-Shannon Professor, Department of Philosophy Denison University, Denison, Ohio

David Wasserman, J.D., M.A., Director of Research, Center for Ethics, Yeshiva University, New York, New York

Preface

A wide swath of contemporary social debates features what might be called "appeals to nature"—claims that nature or a natural state of affairs possesses some special value that should be weighed in moral decision-making and perhaps protected in public policy. These appeals are of a variety of kinds and involve many different understandings of what "nature" means. While none of them fit easily into the classical accounts of moral values in Western moral philosophy, they have enduring power in everyday moral discussion and, recently, somewhat wider acceptance in the scholarly literature, giving them significant clout in a range of contemporary social debates.

Perhaps the most prominent of these debates is over what humans may do to themselves and to others—from the kinds of relationships they may form with each other to the biotechnological interventions by means of which they can actually change their own or their children's bodies. Concerns about which human relationships are "natural" have a long history rooted chiefly in religiously oriented natural law traditions; however, a range of commentators have recently developed concerns in a more expressly secular fashion about how biotechnology might change the very categories of nature, including the category of human nature. The President's Council on Bioethics, formed by President Bush in August 2001 to address the ethical and policy ramifications of biomedical innovation, argued against a variety of biotechnological alterations of human bodies and human practices on grounds that the changes would be "dehumanizing" (President's Council on Bioethics, 2003). From a very different political perspective, the environmentalist Bill McKibben followed up his book *The End of Nature* with *Enough,* which lamented that human genetic engineering and other technologies will bring about "the end of human nature" (McKibben, 2003). The communitarian political philosopher Michael Sandel argues that the "deeper danger" in using gene transfer technologies to enhance ourselves or our children is that doing so represents "a Promethean impulse" to remake nature, including human nature, that inappropriately elevates human willfulness and mastery (Sandel, 2007, pp. 89ff.). It is widely (though certainly not universally) held that athletes should not be permitted to use performance-enhancing drugs. And people of a variety of viewpoints hold that we should die natural deaths, not planned ones carried out with a doctor's assistance, and not ones indefinitely postponed by means of tomorrow's "antiaging" technologies.

Another category of high-profile social debates that feature appeals to nature concerns other species. This category includes debates about agricultural bio-technology and what might be called "pet biotechnology"—such as the develop-ment of a fish, originally created for industrial purposes but now marketed as a pet, that glows red or green in the dark. These appeals to nature are frequently subordinated to other moral concerns, that agricultural biotechnology will have bad environmental consequences or bad consequences for human health and well-being, for instance. Much of the argument against genetically modified corn, for example, focuses on whether it might kill off monarch butterflies. The language in these debates, however—coining terms such as "Frankenfood" and "Monsatan" (playing on the name of the company, Monsanto, a leading producer of genetically modified seeds)—suggests that those opposed to biotechnology think the problem is something ungodly, something reminiscent of Dr. Franken-stein. At times the appeal to nature emerges openly. Some European philosophers have argued, for example, that genetically modifying chickens to become insen-tient egg producers would unacceptably violate their "species integrity," even though it would benefit humans and possibly even chickens (Bovenkerk, Brom, and van den Bergh, 2002). When the California Fish and Game Commission de-cided to ban the "Glo-fish," one commissioner told a reporter with the *San Fran-cisco Chronicle,* "At the end of the day, I don't think it's right to produce a new or-ganism just to be a pet. What's next? A pig with wings? . . . Welcome to the future. Here we are, playing with the genetic bases of life" (Martin, 2003).

In recent years, some argue, the tools and information available for genetically modifying organisms have progressed to the point that the goals have grown much more ambitious and the very identity of the field has changed. Instead of making just a few genetic modifications to existing organisms, and doing so in a largely trial-and-error fashion, we can aim to synthesize entire genomes, then to design basic, simplified genomes and an assortment of genetic "parts," as it were, that code for particular biological functions and that could be assembled in vari-ous combinations and installed in the genome. The product of this genetic con-struction would be a synthetic organism, and the work of producing it has been dubbed "synthetic biology." The near-term goals of synthetic biology are microbes specially engineered to produce medicines or fuels. Still, the question has been raised whether in going from genetic modification to synthetic biology the human relationship to nature has changed "from 'manipulatio' to 'creatio ex existendo'" (Boldt and Müller, 2008).

When the argument against agricultural biotechnology rests on a concern about its effect on the natural world, it may amount to an indirect appeal to nature, for the environment is the focus of a third category of debates involving appeals to nature. As in debates about agricultural biotechnology, appeals to nature in environmental disputes take the form of claims about what is natural for nonhuman entities, in this case about the patterns and diversity of species, wildernesses, ecosystems, and other natural phenomena. If debates about medical biotechnology involve claims about human nature, and debates about agricultural biotechnology involve claims about nonhuman nature in human settings, then environmentalism is about nonhuman nature in isolation from human beings.

In the environmental domain, unlike debates about animal and medical biotechnology, appeals to nature have clearly led to policy. The Endangered Species Act of 1973, for example, arguably presupposes that species ought to be preserved for their own sake—or, more accurately, that species ought to be protected from human endangerment for their own sakes and allowed to go extinct only through natural causes. Many of the species in whose interests the act is invoked do not provide significant benefit for humankind—not enough to outweigh the benefits of the hunting, fishing, logging, or recreational activity that threatens them. The anger and indignation environmentalists feel about species loss seem to reflect an underlying concern about the species themselves, a sense that it is simply wrong, at least in the absence of strong countervailing considerations, to cause naturally occurring forms of life to disappear from the world. Likewise, the Wilderness Act of 1964 appears to presuppose the intrinsic value of spaces that are, in the language of the act, "untrammeled by man." If they are untrammeled, then relatively few people are directly benefiting from their preservation, and the moral rationale for their preservation seems to lie in something other than human benefit. Again, in the debate over logging old-growth forests, the problem with logging them all cannot be just the loss of a valuable resource: not to log them is also to lose the resource. Similar impulses may lie behind the creation of the federal national park system.

A Comparative Examination of Appeals to Nature

A spate of scholarly and popular books, reports, and articles has advanced arguments of one sort or another about appeals to nature, but sustained comparative studies that take on the entire range of appeals to nature are rare. Instead, these writings have tended to remain within the confines of a particular subject—environmental ethics, where "nature" is central to debates about what should be protected (or sometimes, restored); agricultural ethics, where the concept of "nature" has been invoked and criticized in debates about genetically modified crops and livestock; and bioethics, which includes issues of medical biotechnology and its use to enhance human nature. This volume of essays, emerging from a three-year research project conducted by the Hastings Center and funded by the National Endowment for the Humanities, tries to advance thinking about "nature" in a more broadly comparative fashion. The project took up the three broad social debates identified above—about human nature, about domesticated organisms, and about the preservation and protection of the environment. The essays in this volume have more to say about human nature and the use of medical enhancement—the Hastings Center's home turf—than about the other topics, but all of them are informed by other debates, some engage in explicitly comparative work, and as a group they seek to set work in other domains, especially concerning the environment, alongside work in bioethics.

Three broad questions animated the project. The first is a question of conceptual clarification: What does "nature" or "natural" mean? What are the similarities and differences across different social debates in how the idea of "nature" is deployed? The second is a question in moral philosophy: If a state of affairs is natural, can its being natural ever have any moral significance? Can its being natural be valued *for that reason alone,* not merely because it helps show how to achieve some other morally valuable end? Do the different uses of "nature" function similarly? The third question moves from moral to political philosophy: May appeals to nature affect public policy? If so, are they moral trump cards, or should they be fitted in alongside or weighed against other moral concerns?

Consensus is almost unimaginable on these questions, and the contributors to this volume do not seek it. The goal is rather to turn the issues in the light for a while. Some of the contributors return to and refine the critique of "nature" that goes back to John Stuart Mill. Others look to defend appeals to nature. Among those that attempt a defense, however, opinions cluster in suggestive ways—revealing

not a consensus, but at least a constellation of related opinions, and perhaps opening up promising avenues for further work.

With respect to the first, conceptual set of questions, for example, a theme link-
ing several chapters is that while "nature" and "human nature" elude clear definitions, clear definitions may also not be necessary. Several papers also consider
the possibility that the concepts of "nature" and "human nature" can be considered in relatively narrow and metaphysically modest ways. A couple of papers
explore the possibility that "nature" might refer only to the nature of a species
rather than to a special "essence" of a species or to a broad ontological distinction
between what is natural and what is artificial. Several also consider the possibility
that the understanding of nature might even be, in some part, a social construct.

Similarly, with respect to the second kind of questions—those about the moral
significance of "the natural"—several of the chapters defending appeals to nature
explore the possibility that "naturalness" might make only a limited moral difference. In particular, a distinction between natural and not natural need not point
to a general distinction between permissible and impermissible to have moral significance. Instead of a general distinction, several papers propose, the distinction
might be specific to a given context, such as sports. Or, following a line developed
in some other papers, instead of outlining the limits of the permissible, appeals to
nature might seek to ground only an attitude of humility or of respect and forbearance, not sufficient to prevent all human interference in natural states of affairs but
enough to generate misgivings about frivolous destruction of nature.

The third set of questions, about the intersection of moral concerns with the
political sphere, is taken up explicitly only toward the end of the volume, but
again the theme is that a qualified, limited role can be allotted to appeals to
nature. The connection between moral claims and public policy in a democratic
society is more complicated than those who write mostly about the moral claims
sometimes recognize. In many cases, this question, which is a matter of political
philosophy more than of moral philosophy, is left unaddressed entirely. The assumption seems to be that if supporters secure the moral claims about appeals to
nature, then the public policy will follow automatically. In fact, moral positions
should not always be reflected in public policy, and when they do they might be
reflected only indirectly—sometimes, for example, a democratically elected government should merely preserve the possibility that citizens can act on their
moral positions, either individually or in private associations. In the case of
sports, it might be accomplished (to at least some extent) by allowing decisions

about policy concerning athletic enhancement to devolve to privately run sports-governing bodies. Also, as the last chapter in this volume argues, the regulation of biotechnological enhancement may sometimes fall outside the realm of basic social justice; when it does, the values to which regulators appeal may not need to meet the same standards for universal public acceptance that applies to matters of basic social justice.

Organization of the Volume

The chapters are organized roughly according to how they take up these three questions, with earlier chapters focusing on conceptual problems and later chapters bringing greater attention to moral and political concerns—although discussions in each chapter cut across all these questions to some degree. The chapters are also divided between those that consider older work in the Western philosophical canon on the moral relevance of nature and human nature, and those that consider contemporary problems invoking appeals to nature ; the more historically oriented chapters come toward the beginning of the volume.

In the opening chapter, Kate Soper discusses a range of social debates in which the concept of nature appears, and she introduces the problems and tensions inherent in deploying the concept and in jettisoning it. She endorses a certain skepticism about nature, arguing that attempts to clearly delineate "naturality" are largely unsatisfying and that the concept of nature by itself is of little use in practical reasoning because whether something is natural does not by itself tell us what to do. At the same time, she underscores how difficult it is to exclude appeals to nature, and she observes that a flat dismissal of *any* way of understanding the concept would lead to incoherent idealism. She seeks to recapture a "realist concept of nature," which she argues "is indispensable to the coherence both of ecological discourses about the 'changing face of nature,' conceived as a surface environment, and to any discourse about the genetically engineered or cultural 'construction' of human beings or their bodies."

Soper draws on a wide assortment of thinkers in the Western philosophical tradition. Chapters 2 and 3 continue this effort, looking for a defensible and nuanced concept of nature in historical resources. In chapter 2, Jean Porter argues that the early scholastic conception of natural law is relevant (surprisingly enough, she admits) to contemporary concerns about nature and the human relationship to it. The scholastic concept of natural law was friendly to the idea of nature and optimistic about the capacities of the human intellect to understand and appropriately value the natural world. Reflecting a robust philosophy of nature that began to emerge in the late eleventh century and a broadly expansive and open theology emphasizing the intrinsic intelligibility and goodness of the created order, the scholastic idea of nature points suggests new ways of thinking about human alteration of the natural world. It also, argues Porter, identifies possible common ground in the contemporary debate between religion and science.

In chapter 3, Bruce Jennings explores the role of nature and human nature in the early development of social contract theory—the dominant line of thought about social obligation and authority. Jennings argues that Hobbes and Rousseau gave discourse about human nature the fundamental place in their cultural theories. Their conception of nature, however, is independent of any metaphysic, cosmology, or theology and leaves it to human beings to construct cultural order without any transcendent pattern to follow—they assert that universal rational principles provide no definitive guidance; nor is there divine inspiration to be followed.

The next three chapters focus on how the concept of "natural" is used in specific debates. In chapter 4, Gregory E. Kaebnick considers the concept of "human nature" and asks what philosophical commitments about human nature are implied by a moral objection to altering human nature. He proposes that some positions require very well-developed and inflexible understandings of human nature but that others can be much looser, and even incomplete, contrary to what many commentators believe. In particular, he draws a contrast between positions requiring an "essentialist" understanding of human nature and those that do not. In developing his argument, he sets out a taxonomy of positions on the concept of human nature and its moral significance.

Chapters 5 and 6 turn to the use of "nature" in debates about environmental protection and preservation. Eric Katz offers the most unbending defense of "nature" in the volume. He asserts that there is a real ontological difference between natural entities and artifacts and that "nature" is a significant moral category for the development of public policy. "Maintaining this distinction," he argues, "serves as a check on the arrogant notion that human power and human knowledge is unlimited, that human science and technology is capable of dominating and controlling the entire world." Without it, he fears, we will awake one day to a fully humanized world. "This will be a world of parks, but not of wilderness. It will be a world of playing fields, but not of meadows, a world of canals and waterways, but not of rivers."

In chapter 6, Steven Vogel offers a counterpoint to Katz, with a thorough rejection of the concept of "nature." Vogel argues for a "postnaturalist" environmental philosophy—a philosophy after the end of "nature." He argues that it is needed because nature might already have ended and because we do not really know what nature *is,* or how and why to distinguish it from the human. The concept of "nature" is so ambiguous and problematic, "so prone to misunderstanding and so riddled with pitfalls, that its usefulness for a coherent environmental philosophy will turn out to be small indeed."

Katz closes his discussion of "nature" by trying to extend his work, grounded in environmental philosophy, to questions concerning the human relationship to *human* nature. Chapters 7 and 8 carry this comparative challenge forward. Starting with the critique of "nature" found in John Stuart Mill (a critique that also underlies Vogel's analysis), Bonnie Steinbock sorts through a variety of contemporary ways of discussing the human relationship to nature. She argues that many influential contemporary conceptions of nature are inadequate, but she concludes that moral concerns about nature can have moral weight. Factual claims about nature can justify caution about the use of new technologies. Moreover, our humility and awe when confronted with the power and beauty of nature are appropriate and suggest that reducing nature to its commercial value is crass. We should feel gratitude for the natural world, Steinbock argues, but we should not blindly accept nature as a guide for our actions, nor should we reject something simply on the grounds that it does not exist in nature.

Paul Lauritzen writes about the idea of gratitude as well, but from a literary angle. He draws on the work of novelist Cormac McCarthy and essayist Wendell Berry to argue that the need to cultivate certain virtues, especially humility, often stands behind appeals to nature. Much of Lauritzen's work has been on the use of medical biotechnology; in chapter 9 he broadens his focus to include agricultural biotechnology and environmentalism. Like Steinbock, he looks for a plausible, halfway position on "nature"—a way of understanding the concept that gives it moral heft but does not turn it into an inflexible, overriding moral requirement. He writes that, at least in McCarthy's and Berry's thought, altering nature does not look to be intrinsically wrong, nor does it always generate unacceptable consequences. We should nonetheless attempt it only with a sense of caution and humility, acknowledging "our ignorance and our misplaced pride."

Human enhancement in the context of sports provides useful case studies for thinking about appeals to nature. It also, as Nicholas Agar notes, could set a powerful precedent for appeals to nature in other domains. The concluding four chapters focus on appeals to "the natural" in the context of sports, reprising all of the questions that have been broached in previous chapters. In chapter 9, David Wasserman offers a generally critical assessment of objections grounded in the concept of "nature" to biotechnological enhancement of athletes. He argues that it is difficult to develop a coherent and morally defensible account of "the natural" in sports and hard to predict how sports might be altered as enhancements creep in. He concludes that the concept of "the natural" might yet be resuscitated as referring not strictly to a divide between natural and artificial but to one between different practices that either respect or violate the background conditions framing the way the competition is understood and the meaning and value it has for participants and spectators. Practices that respect widely accepted and well-established conditions are deemed "natural," and innovative practices that challenge these conditions, and may challenge the meaning found in the competition, appear to be "unnatural."

In chapter 10, Agar argues forcefully for a restrictive stance toward human enhancement in sports. His appeal is to the interests of spectators. Spectators want to watch sporting performances that are not only exceptional but also produced by competitors similar to them in ways they care about. Performance-enhancing drugs and genetic modifications offend against this sense of shared humanity. Sports are a kind of drama, Agar suggests. To play Hamlet well, it is not enough to remember every line perfectly and enter and exit the stage on cue. One must convey Hamlet's humanity to the audience.

Employing what he calls the "common-sense morality" developed and deployed by Aristotle—an approach that focuses on examples, draws out concepts, definitions, and principles as possible but accepts, if necessary, fuzzier demarcations and family resemblances—William Galston attempts in chapter 11 to show how the distinction between therapy and enhancement can be useful in thinking through the ethics of human enhancements. Although the distinction does not permit one to draw a line between what is permitted and forbidden, it "points to a structure of justification." Enhancement serves goals, Galston argues, whose validity and importance must be assessed case by case. He develops some presumptive principles about which kinds of performance-oriented enhancements are justified and which are not.

The volume concludes with a discussion of sports enhancement that considers, at length, the political significance of appeals to nature—specifically, the place of appeals to human nature in a Rawlsian framework. Thomas H. Murray and Peter Murray argue that John Rawls's theory of justice not only carves out a space in moral and political debate for ideas about human nature but also serves as a model for how to generate conceptions of human nature that could serve as normatively important ideals. They argue that John Rawls, "unsurpassed philosopher of justice and lover of baseball," helps us understand the place of sport and of the concept of "natural talents" in a liberal society.

Although the scope of the volume is very broad, many interesting topics are not addressed in it. For example, the relatively new topic of synthetic biology, mentioned above, is not expressly treated, although general categories of questions raised here—about how the concept "nature" is understood, whether and how that concept legitimately figures in moral discourse, and whether and how moral discourse about it legitimately figures in political discourse—are all relevant for thinking about synthetic biology. Synthetic biology raises these questions in a particularly fundamental form, since it broaches the related conceptual question "What is life?" and the related moral question "What is the proper human relationship to life?" Even supposing that humans may *modify* existing living things, the further question arises whether they may create entirely new forms of life, as some strands of synthetic biology seek to do. There are also reasons for thinking that synthetic biology poses less of a challenge to the human relationship to nature than some other kinds of interventions, including genetic modification (of crops and livestock), on which synthetic biology is a technical advance. Synthetic biology is not yet about crops and livestock; it is only about microbes—not exactly the most charismatic of species and not at the forefront of most environmentalists' concerns. Discussing synthetic biology would require an examination of the particular way it raises concerns about the human relationship to nature; nonetheless, the essays here should at least provide a leg up with that further work.

The very old topic of sex—the original synthetic biology, perhaps—is also not treated. The questions at the intersection of sex, nature, and morality are various, of course. They include, for starters, questions about sexual relationships, familial and other relationships between the sexes, the role of sex within the family, and the implications of artificial reproductive technologies. Again, the three general categories of questions broached here are relevant, but again, particular issues would also have to be taken up. For example, to talk about sexual relationships, it would not be enough to know generally how to handle the concept of "nature"; we would also need to have a lot of information about what actually *is* natural. There are important factual questions at stake—more than could be adequately handled in this volume. Additionally, we would have to consider whether it is general types that we are interested in or individual cases. That is, would a belief that the human relationship to nature is morally significant translate into a belief that statistical norms about human beings generate value norms to which people ought to try to conform, or is the point rather that we ought to cherish even natural diversity? This point is taken up briefly in Kaebnick's essay.

Some ways of thinking about "nature" are also left out of the volume. For example, although several of the discussions emphasize Aristotelian reasoning, an extended discussion of Aristotelian lines of thought is not included. Nothing in the volume draws exclusively on religious traditions either. The "deep ecology" movement, whose adherents argue that nature has an especially strong kind of intrinsic value (significant in its own right, rather than merely as a way of achieving other ends, and existing independently of whether anybody recognizes that value) is also not represented. To some degree, these omissions reflect the fact that the volume comes out of two meetings held at the Hastings Center in 2006 and 2007. In some cases, they also reflect a decision to concentrate on perspectives that try to avoid relatively extreme or narrowing metaphysical commitments—claims about the nature of the cosmos, that is, that make that perspective interesting chiefly within a particular tradition. The goal has been to think about moral attitudes toward nature within a secular and fairly mainstream space of reasons and to think critically but constructively about what might be said about them. What has emerged is a predictably wide range of opinions, but within that range an intriguing constellation of positions that defend appeals to nature. These positions are united by the loose theme that there might be qualified, limited ways of understanding appeals to nature that allow them to play a role in individual moral positions, and perhaps even in public policy, but do not carve out a decisive role for them.

REFERENCES

Boldt, J., and O. Müller. 2008. "Newtons of the Leaves of Grass." *Nature Biotechnology* 26:387–89.
Bovenkerk, B., F. W. A. Brom, and B. J. van den Bergh. 2002. "Brave New Birds: The Use of 'Animal Integrity' in Animal Ethics." *Hastings Center Report* 32 (1): 16–22.
Martin, M. 2003. "Glowing Fish? When Pigs Fly, State Says." *San Francisco Chronicle*, December 4.

McKibben, B. 2003. *Enough: Genetic Engineering and the End of Human Nature.* London: Bloomsbury.

President's Council on Bioethics. 2003. *Beyond Therapy: Biotechnology and the Pursuit of Happiness.* Washington, D.C.

Sandel, M., 2007. *The Case against Perfection: Ethics in the Age of Genetic Engineering.* Cambridge, Mass.: Belknap Press of Harvard University Press.

The Ideal of Nature

CHAPTER ONE

Disposing Nature or Disposing of It?

Reflections on the Instruction of Nature

Kate Soper, M.A.

In the well-known maxim "Culture proposes, Nature disposes," it is implied that we humans may have hypotheses about the ways that nature works but that nature itself will settle the issue. The question at hand is precisely whether the invocation of nature to decide questions of environmental or biomedical policy can finally settle anything. On what grounds can we reasonably discriminate between activities and interventions in terms of their "naturality"—and what is the normative burden of doing so? Does X being determined as "natural" render it either more generally acceptable or morally compelling; if so, why? In short, does "nature" instruct us in any universally agreeable sense on what we should do, or not do, either to ourselves or our management of the environment? Can it figure as a moral ideal we should choose to uphold, at least in some contexts? Or is it the case, as Steven Vogel (2006) claimed, that we should be better off disposing with any reference to it altogether? In short, does nature dispose, or should we dispose of it?

Thirty years ago, these questions would hardly have been addressed in the academy. Or if they had been, they would have been broached for the most part to challenge spurious claims about the supposed "perversity" of homosexuality or about the "naturally" ordained character of divisions and differences (relating to class, gender, ethnicity) that in reality owed more to social construction than to biological determination. It was, in short, to undermine reactionary attempts to invoke "nature" as a means of policing behavior (especially sexual behavior) or of perpetuating—by presenting them as "natural" and thus as immutable—dimensions of existence that were in reality socially instituted. The challenge, as Jonathan Dollimore and others have pointed out, was to the "violence" done in the name of "nature" rather than to the offenses caused by its dismissal (Dollimore, 1991, pp. 114–15; Soper, 1995, pp. 119–48, esp. 145 n.2). Most of these objectors were left-leaning and saw their interventions as a progressive response to regrettable forms of social conservatism or even bigotry.

In that intellectual context, the quarrel—to invoke the distinction developed by Gregory Kaebnick in this volume—was with the use of "nature" as a group norm in policing individual behavior, and the appeal to nature was thought of as an appeal to an ontological fixity whose "endorsement" would guarantee the unalterable quality of whatever was stamped as "natural." Hence, the usage became problematic in discussions about class, gender, and race. Today, antifoundationalist theories, most influentially the arguments of Foucault and his followers, have challenged earlier conceptions of the "natural," which signified givens of biology or physics, seeing such conceptions instead as inherently revisable cultural norms. (Foucault and his arguments have also been influential around the idea of the "reverse discourse" in encouraging individuals to resist not only the oppression of supposedly natural group norms but also any approving redescription of their alleged individual "perversity" as, in fact, "equally natural.")[1]

There have also been dramatic developments in genetic engineering and other technical advances that have removed many of the earlier, biologically based determinants of social policy and practice. Our developed powers over "nature" in recent decades have led us to be more often at the mercy of what culture and economic and social policy enforces than to be subject to biological dictates. It is easier to obtain breast enhancement and other forms of cosmetic surgery than it is to shift stereotypes of beauty and sexual attraction. Much of the illness and misery afflicting the world's poorest could be eradicated were it not for the economic relations and political orders standing in the way. It is, in other words, often simpler to counter and alter what is genetically determined than to curb or transform the conventions of culture (Soper, 1995, pp. 139–40). We have also witnessed the massive erosion and exhaustion of environmental territory and resources that ecologists often call the "loss," or even the "end," of nature. The practical and theoretical impact of these developments is becoming more apparent. Growing concerns voiced across the political spectrum, by no means confined to its more reactionary elements, raise questions about "unnatural" activity of various kinds, including humanly wrought transformations of the natural environment and the hugely enhanced powers of biotechnology.

Over recent decades, then, we have seen a considerable shift of normative emphasis and the emergence of a whole spectrum of nature-endorsing or pro-naturalist discourses, motivated by the prospect of the "end" or "death" of nature and concerned with rescuing nature from its socialization and presenting it as the constraint on or counter to constructivist understandings and forms of complacency. From this side of things, the concern is less to expose false forms of naturalization of the social than to discover whether "nature" might still provide an ontological basis or ultimate court of appeal for condemning a whole range of existing practices both in everyday production and consumption and in science and genetics (genetically modified foods, cloning, nanotechnology, new drug therapies, the use of recreational drugs, and so forth). Such practices are "not natural," people protest. But instead of right-wing ideologues railing against same-sex relations, women boxing, or other supposed perversities, the cry comes from those (including many on the left) who are keen to protect us from what they see as abusive and false forms of progress. Members of the public often register similar protests against the more intrusive applications of biotechnology.

The most explicit concerns about new scientific development and biotechnical interventions—both of experts and of the public at large—are usually those to do with success, utility, and safety. In the United Kingdom's response to foods produced through genetic modification (GM), the main questions asked were whether crop enhancement and protection of non-GM agriculture could be achieved in the way pro-GM scientists claimed, whether GM production was expedient or necessary to achieve the ends proposed, and, perhaps above all, whether it could be guaranteed to be safe in both human and ecological terms. Much conflicting scientific evidence was submitted in the disputes. There has also been justified concern about the immorality of the huge profits made by GM companies. But underlying these concerns—and influencing the reception and interpretation of the scientific data offered for or against such developments as GM—has been a concern with the counter-naturality of the process. Are such developments a step too far in the manipulation of nature, a hubristic affront to what one might call our moral sense of what humans may properly do with their powers of intervention? The notion of "Frankenstein science" often invoked in this context indicates this revulsion. (See, for example, the evidence cited by Kaebnick, 2007, including in the United States, despite the generally more tolerant attitude to GM there than in Europe.)[2]

As other chapters in this volume note, however, such a response raises other questions. On what grounds are we determining the "naturality" of such new developments, and how, if at all, do they differ from earlier human constructions of or interactions with nature? What is the criterion of the "natural" at work here, and how coherent is it? Traditionally, "natural" production has been distinguished from "artificial" by its undeliberated, preprogrammed, or instinctual character. This is certainly the basis of Immanuel Kant's influential discriminations in his *Critique of Judgment*. There he tells us that what differentiates the naturally produced object from the artistic or artifactual is the lack of a deliberated intention to create it (1987, p. 170). Because the productions of other animals are instinctual and preprogrammed, there is neither the conscious intentionality to produce a certain kind of entity nor the reflective meditation on its achievement that mark human productions as artifacts or works of art. But in the division of the *Critique* titled "Analytical of Teleological Judgment" (pp. 373–75), Kant also insists that organisms such as plants and animals are uniquely distinctive in being natural purposes; that is, they are organized as wholes in which all the parts combine into a unity and operate reciprocally as cause and effect of their form (p. 252). A natural organism is what we might term a self-occurring and self-generating entity, or as Kant puts it, an entity that is both cause and effect of itself. In this, he indicates, it differs profoundly both from a painting or work of literature but also from a mechanism such as a watch:

> In a watch one part is the instrument which makes the others move, but one gear is not the efficient cause that produces another gear; [and hence] even though one part is there for the sake of another, the former part is not there as a result of the latter. That is also the reason why the cause that produced the watch and its form does not lie in nature (the nature of this material), but lies outside nature and in a being who can act according to the ideas of a whole that he can produce through his causality. It is also the reason why one gear in the watch does not produce another; still less does one watch produce other watches, [by] using (and organizing) other matters for this [production]. It is also the reason why, if parts are removed from the watch, it does not replace them on its own; nor, if parts were missing from it when it was first built, does it compensate for this [lack] by having the other parts help out, let alone repair itself on its own when out of order; yet all of this we can expect organized nature to do. (p. 253)

This organization "strictly speaking . . . has nothing analogous to any causality known to us." The intrinsic natural perfection possessed by organisms, that is, things that are only possible as natural purposes, "is not conceivable or explicable on any analogy to any known physical ability, i.e. ability of nature, not even—since we too belong to nature in the broadest sense—on a precisely fitting analogy to human art" (p. 254). Natural organisms, in other words, cannot be understood either as "intended" by an external agent (as in the case of art) or as mechanistic. (Thus, in his transcendental argument, Kant tells us that what is presupposed in their case is an intuition—which only reason can think—of an understanding of a "whole that makes possible the character and combination of its parts.")

Suggestive as these discriminations are, it is debatable whether they provide much help distinguishing between, for example, more or less natural plant or animal modifications. GM seems plainly artifactual on Kant's criterion insofar as it involves a deliberate intention to produce a certain type of entity, one that would not have come about without that external causality. (Although it is also, of course, to be distinguished from art because the rules for its production can be taught—the scientist just has to follow a given set of procedures.) Yet, once produced, a genetically modified organism has a life and generative force of its own and, thus, a natural purpose in Kant's sense. Similar, if not identical, observations can be made regarding conventional forms of plant breeding and hybridization, the only difference being that these do not rely on the laboratory to the same degree. (Kant presents grafting as if it were part of natural process in section 371). Perhaps, then, the most that could be said is that GM is more artificial—or mechanistic—because it involves more contrivance and relies on bringing together parts within a whole and setting up causal reactions that could never have obtained through more conventional means. This "minimalist" line would also be consistent with those who argue that we cannot expect a sharply defined category of the "natural" in these contexts and that what counts when it comes to claims about "naturality" is not human interference but the degree of its "dominance" or intrusiveness.[3]

It may be said that this type of reaction fudges the point because it does not address the sense that a process like GM is absolutely different from other procedures and interventions and, consequently, "unnatural." But is it? To those who contend that by putting fish genes into strawberries we are breaching the "species barrier," the Nuffield Council's *Report on Genetic Modification* argues that this only raises questions about what constitutes a fish gene (which, it points out, some would say is no more than a defined stretch of DNA in a fish cell). The report also asks whether a plant is "acceptably natural or organic if it has been successively bred to have a particular gene complement, but unnatural and not 'organic' if precisely the same gene complement has been arrived at through laboratory process" (1999, p. 39). And it concludes, perhaps reasonably enough, that there is no reason in ethics to draw a distinction. (Robert Streiffer, 2003, offers the countering argument that the occurrence of gene flow between species in nature does not mean it is natural for humans to move genes between species. Yet the problem here is to decide what, if anything, we can mean by "natural for humans" in the first place.)

It would, then, appear difficult to specify the criteria of naturality that make such examples of biotechnology plainly and uncontroversially "unnatural." Even if it were not, why should the "unnaturality" of certain practices be grounds for opposing them any more than it is grounds to oppose, say, artistic production? After all, GM and similarly advanced biotechnological processes are plainly unnatural according to one of the commonest definitions of the natural (and one invoked by many recent ecological writers), where the kernel idea is that nature is that which is "uncontaminated" by humans or in which humans have had no hand. But then so, too, are most of our other practices, even the least instrumental and unintrusive, because there is nothing that we humans have a hand in shaping or directing that is not unnatural on these grounds. Moreover, many of the medical and environmental interventions generally welcomed uncontroversially as beneficial are extremely "unnatural" on that criterion. So even if we were to agree to some criteria that allowed us to specify which applications of biotechnology are "unnatural" (and, as indicated, this seems difficult to do in any absolute sense), it is by no means clear that anything much would hang thereby.

Other contributors to this volume also point to the difficulties of deriving an essentialist definition of "nature" that could be used to distinguish between "natural" or "unnatural" practices (whether it be to applaud or reject them). Vogel (2006), for example, is forthright in dismissing the idea that any helpful discriminations can be made through the concept. He argues that not only "might nature the thing have ended[,] the *concept* of 'nature' might be such an ambiguous and problematic one, so prone to misunderstanding and so riddled with pitfalls, that its usefulness for a coherent environmental philosophy might be small indeed."

Even though Vogel is right, in my opinion, about the problems of invoking nature in any moral sense, he is too ready to elide the dismissal of "nature" with the rejection of *any* concept of nature at all. For there is *one* sense in which nature does always "dispose," or have its say in human activities, and this is the sense in which all our interventions, whether environmental or biological in respect of ourselves or other beings, depend on the workings of physical law and process and have their outcomes determined by them. In making this point, I am invoking what I and others influenced by Critical Realism have argued is the difference between a "realist" or theoretical concept of nature and other more phenomenological or metaphysical concepts (Benton, 1989, 1992; Soper, 1995, pp. 149–76; Soper, 1996). Nature in the "realist" sense refers us to structures and processes independent of human activity (in the sense that they are not humanly created) and whose forces and causal powers are the condition of, and constraint on, any human practice, however ambitious (genetic engineering, the creation of new energy sources, attempted manipulations of the climate, attempts to "terraform" other planets, or any other Promethean scheme). This is the "nature" to whose laws we are always subject, even as we harness them to human purposes, and whose processes we can neither escape nor destroy. This is the "nature" that cannot be said to be "ending" whatever we do to planet Earth, because it will persist in its workings even in the midst of nuclear holocaust or destruction by asteroid or solar combustion.

This realist concept of nature, I have argued in *What Is Nature?* (1995), is indispensable to the coherence both of ecological discourses about the "changing face of nature," conceived as a surface environment, and of any discourse about the genetically engineered or cultural "construction" of human beings or their bodies. Environmental transformations, whether we deem them malign or benign and whether humanly designed (ancient barrow, nuclear bunker, or nature park) or not (earthquake, volcano, tsunami), require us to distinguish between their "nature," in the sense of pregiven powers and processes at work in their creation, and their more empirically observable (and humanly useful or damaging) environmental effects. In the same fashion, we must recognize the natural body or physiological process as a condition of any controlling intervention or cultural work on it, no matter whether voluntary or coerced, or however profound and intrusive in its alterations. I previously have made this point in reference to the so-called construction of gender and sexuality, arguing that emphasis on the variable and culturally relative quality of human sexuality requires, as its counterpart, recognition of the more constant and universal features of embodied existence if it is to be meaningful. But the same points apply to any form of medical bioengineering, given its reliance on the "natural" laws and processes of human biology.

Admittedly, nature in this realist sense carries no normative weight. It may, indeed, "dispose" us in a scientific-technical sense for or against certain types of action, and it will always have its say in determining their effects, but it does not endorse any particular way of living or being. Regarding the environment, nature may exercise an influence on what we do, or can even try to do, but we have to decide what it is ethical to attempt within those limits. Likewise, as biological organisms, we have certain requirements or instinctual responses that we cannot resist (to breathe, digest, excrete), but there is also a range of biological needs and influences that are subject to extensive manipulation and cultural mediation and in that sense not wholly determining on any individual's behavior. Even in the case of a "basic" need such as that for food, the individual can decide to resist it—and does so in cases of anorexia or voluntary fasting. Heterosexual relations, which have been presented in some gender theory, as an arbitrary and even coercive norm of human sexual conduct (Rich, 1983; Butler, 1990, 1993; Jeffreys, 1990), are a prescription of nature in the sense that they have been essential to the reproduction of the species. Yet it is in principle possible today to circumvent the contacts between the sexes involved in reproduction of this kind, and were we to make an ethicopolitical decision to do so, "realist" nature would not step in to prevent us. In making this option, however, we would not escape the determination of biology. On the contrary, we would need to know an awful lot about it to commit to such a scenario (Soper, 1996, pp. 31–32).

If, then, the theorists who tell us "there is no nature" are denying its reality and specific determinations in this understanding, then they are committed to a form of idealism that is incoherent. I take it, therefore, that when writers such as Bill McKibben or Carolyn Merchant speak of the "end" or "death" of nature, or insist (like Vogel) that we have now moved to a "postnature" condition, they are not denying the continuation of nature in this sense.

As we have seen, however, nature in this realist sense cannot exercise more than a limited determination on our choices and remains normatively indifferent to them. Nor does it seem possible to identify any other concept of "nature" that can more successfully supply us with an ethics. Perhaps, then, we should give up on any attempt to do so and adopt, as Kaebnick suggested, a more Wittgensteinian approach that reflects on usage rather than seeking to police it? Indeterminacy, Kaebnick (2008) suggests, does not render the concept of "nature" unserviceable. On the contrary, it can help to make a point about the degree or kind of human intervention in given situations: "It need not be an all-or-nothing case, nor need there even be any precise rule about what degree or kind of human intervention makes something 'unnatural,' for the term to be meaningful and useful."

Might we, proceeding in this more particularist spirit, do better to explore what, if anything, is distinctive to moral appeals to nature in specific contexts: to ask, not what makes X "unnatural," but what is peculiar to the opprobrium attaching to the idea that it is and how does it differ from other forms of moral disapproval? Why is it, for example, that we tend to condemn necrophilia and pedophilia as "perverse" or "unnatural" (as well as wrong) but not murder or rape, which we instead denounce simply as "wrong" or "evil"? Is this because we implicitly discriminate between acts that other animals *cannot* do and those they *do not* do? Others animals, of course, kill each other frequently and regularly use force in sexual intercourse, but only humans can murder or rape because these are acts that figure as morally culpable only in the context of the human community. Necrophilia, by contrast, although certainly deemed immoral and criminalized, we also condemn as unnatural—in virtue, it might seem, of its proving the exception to the norm for animal behavior.

Yet it can seem just as problematic to police human behavior by reference to what is "natural" for other animals, as to deal with animals as if they had moral understanding. According to Freud, moreover, the so-called perversions have an "originary" status for human beings, being a given of human nature that has to be repressed as a condition of civilization. "Society," Freud writes, "believes that no greater threat to its civilization could arise than if the sexual instincts were to be liberated and returned to their original aims. For this society does not wish to be reminded of this precarious portion of its foundations" (Freud, 1974–86, 1:48; cf. 7:86; 8:268). He suggests the loathing toward manifest perversions has a similar source: "It is as though one could not forget that they are not only something disgusting but also something monstrous and dangerous—as though people felt them as seductive, and had at bottom to fight down a secret envy of those who were enjoying them" (1:363). Indeed, he presents this disgust with perversions as purely conventional, illogical, and irrational (7:64; 8:83–84). Yet, as Jonathan Dollimore has pointed out, it would be naïve of Freud to expect us to rid ourselves of shame or disgust because these are—as he himself argued (7:76 esp. n.1; 7:75)—the fundamental principles of cultural order (Dollimore, 1991, p. 180).

The "unnatural" or "perverse" in these contexts speak to a species-specific and exclusive need for us to police divisions (between life and death, children and adults, nourishment and excretion, humans and animals) whose maintenance is seen as a condition of the possibility of any human community. In Kaja Silverman's words, perversion "subverts many of the binary oppositions upon which the social order rests: it crosses the boundary separating food from excrement (coprophilia); human from animal (bestiality); life from death (necrophilia); adult from child (pederasty); and pleasure and pain (masochism)" (1988, p. 33).

Obviously, these divisions can be challenged, and they frequently are: posthumanism, of the kind Donna Haraway and other cyborg theorists promote, would move beyond the observance of clear-cut distinctions between humans, animals, and machines (Haraway, 1991, 1997; cf. Hardt and Negri, 2000).[4] But there is also a certain circularity in these arguments given their own reliance on ethical appeal. Haraway calls on us to blur or collapse the animal-human-machine distinctions and embrace instead a cyborg ontology that cheerfully accepts the "leakiness" of these boundaries. But she does so in the name of promoting human sexual emancipation and more humane treatment of animals, and it is difficult to see how such goals can be consistent with the refusal to recognize distinctions between the body and the machine, humans and other animals. Any form of protest against the cruelties of agribusiness and biotechnology is a protest against the treatment of organic beings as if they were mere Cartesian machines indifferent to the sufferings of their flesh; the disembodied cyborg hardly seems the icon to employ in objecting to torture, or indeed to any form of assault on the flesh. Respect for the distinctive pleasures and pains of human love and sexuality is also inconsistent with the erosion of the human-animal divide. Referring us to DuPont's OncoMouse,[5] Haraway tells us that, gazing "from the mutated rodent eyes at her hominid kin," she would raise questions of kinship: how are natural kinds to be identified in the new realm of aliens and transpecifics? "Who," she asks "are my familiars, my siblings, and what kinds of liveable world are we trying to build?" (1997, pp. 51–55). These are, indeed, apposite questions, but that we see them as such, and agonize about the moral dilemmas they pose, is precisely because we still observe our organic-inorganic, human-animal, conceptual divisions. The irony of the invitation to blur these is that if we were truly able to do so, we would no longer recognize the force of the moral problems that Haraway is posing. A world bereft of these distinctions is a world bereft of the grounding conditions of any recognizable form of moral, political, or scientific critique. Is that we may ask, a "liveable world"?

Moreover, even though the appeal to nature is always vexed and troubled, it is difficult to keep it out of the picture altogether. Thus, we find that even those most critical of attempts to provide a criterion of naturality often end up by gesturing toward the idea, if only implicitly. As we have seen, the Nuffield *Report on Genetic Modification* rejects the idea that "nature" can be invoked for or against GM. Yet it simultaneously claims that "naturalness" and "unnaturalness" are part of a spectrum—a point it explicates by reference to more or less conventional methods of plant breeding: "'Naturalness' and 'unnaturalness' are part of a spectrum. At one end of the scale, some modifications of the plants that are now being achieved by genetic modification might also have been achieved over time by conventional means of plant breeding; indeed, this has recently occurred. It would be hard to object to such a modification as a matter of principle as being 'unnatural,' since it would only be using a new and presumably more efficient means of achieving a result that could have been achieved by conventional, more 'natural' means" (1999, p. 123). So conceptually the report's authors do seem happy to invoke *some* sort of criterion of what is more or less "natural" even as they refuse to say why.

Vogel, too, wants us to eschew all discourse on "nature," but he nonetheless defends his "postnaturalism" in the name of avoiding environmental disaster and securing human flourishing. Thus he speaks of the "correct" belief that the effects of human activity over the last two centuries have been "baleful" and "destructive" (2006, p. 5). Yet "destruction" and "disaster" arise only in respect to human values, needs, and commitments to certain lifestyles. Once we have dispensed with any reference to nature, including—as Vogel insists—biological nature, then it is hard to argue that some forms of need or desire satisfaction should take preference. In the very phrase "looming environmental disaster," there is an implication of biological imperatives for survival and minimal flourishing that sits uneasily with Vogel's rejection of any appeal to nature. It also sits uneasily with his criticisms of anthropocentricism. Vogel wants us to give up anthropocentric conceptions, yet there is an inevitable element of anthropocentricism in the idea of environmental "disaster," as it is only human beings who are assumed to be in the position to understand, monitor, and possibly preempt that disaster. In this respect, humanity differs profoundly from other species and should be recognized as doing so. But this difference arises not so much in virtue of some exclusively human power, as Vogel put it, "to move things out of the natural realm" because, in the end, there is no "artificial" production that does not comprise natural materials and is not reliant on natural processes. What our species-specific capacities *do* allow us is a vastly greater external matrix of production and a huge reservoir of nonbiologically inherited forms of learning. These capacities set us apart from other creatures—and they are surely "naturally" distinctive to us, which is to say not "outside" nature but very different in character from the nature of other beings (although all these, of course, have their own species-specific characteristics).

Vogel assumes anthropocentrism has to be both triumphalist (as opposed to realistic about human-animal differences) and committed to an antievolutionary perspective. But the human mind can be theorized as an emergence and still recognized as species-specific and ontologically distinctive.

Let me lastly suggest that there is an aesthetic rationale for the appeal to "nature," reflected in arguments on the aesthetic of nature by thinkers such as Kant and Theodor Adorno. The *Critique of Judgment* is marked throughout by a sense that what we aesthetically respond to in nature is a spontaneous purposiveness independent of human desire—its production of beauty without deliberated design. This surely captures something of what lies in the intuitive objections to many biotechnological interventions, namely, that they are set in motion for entirely instrumental reasons—that there is so little in biotechnology that just happens or comes about independently of human intent. In other words, "unnatural" in aesthetic terms figures as a metaphor of resistance to the cognitive control and instrumental rationality involved in such technical manipulations of human or environmental conditions.

The idea of nature as a counter to commodification and the dominance of our own constructions is also at work in Adorno's *Aesthetic Theory* where he refers to Kant as one of the last philosophers to retain suspicions of artifactuality and the "fallibility of making" (i.e., to value nature over art) and presents himself as reconnecting with a lost tradition of interest in the aesthetic of nature. It is an interest paradoxically lost, Adorno claims, because of the influence exercised by Kant, through his emphasis on human freedom and autonomy, on subsequent idealist aesthetics—the upshot being that nothing came to be treated as worthy of respect that did not owe its existence to the human subject. "Natural beauty," Adorno writes, "vanished from aesthetics thanks to the expanding supremacy of the concept of human freedom and dignity inaugurated by Kant but fully realised by Schiller and Hegel, who transplanted these ethical concepts into aesthetics, with the result that in art, like everywhere else, nothing deserved respect unless it owed its existence to the autonomous subject" (1997, p. 92).

Adorno's approach, however, is much more dialectical than Kant's, and any endorsement of the "immediacy" of nature as a counter to instrumental rationality is tempered by his emphasis on its historicity and cultural mediation. Even as Adorno recognizes the summons of what is spontaneously given and preconceptual in nature, he also acknowledges the extent to which what is discoverable as "beautiful" or "worthy" in virtue of its "naturality" owes its reception as such to culture. Adorno, indeed, is as skeptical about the appeal to nature as he is about the appeal to what is cultural or historical, and he constantly uses each to correct the confident pronouncements of the other.

He is resistant *both* to false and fetishizing forms of the naturalization of history *and* to the "enchantment of history," that is, to any view of history as if it were a form of "mastery" of or "escape" from nature. In fact, he suggests that history creates nature in the negative sense (what he terms "second nature") by delivering us up to new forms of fatedness, the apparent necessities of a given social order and economy. Viewed in this light, capitalist society is itself "natural" or ahistorical because it is committed to the eternal reproduction of its relations of production and commodification. GM, nanotechnology, and other forms of biotechnological appropriations of nature, however innovative, looked at in this optic would be no more than business as usual and thus also "natural" in a pejorative sense because they are simply the latest vehicles for the reproduction of the market society and its profit-making and consumerist objectives.

By contrast, Adorno uses the more positive sense "nature"—or "first nature"—to refer to all forms of concrete, individually existing beings that are mortal or transitory (that is, to both corporeal existence and to the products of labor). In this understanding, nature is the embodiment of history and history the vehicle of nature (Adorno, 1973; cf. Adorno, 2006). We might say, then, that it is manifest both in the productions of biotechnology *and* in the resistance of all those individuals who throughout history may pit themselves against dominant forces and tendencies. In this dimension, partly under the influence of Walter Benjamin, Adorno emphasizes history's "one-timeness." History is a transitory affair from which there is no going back and in and through which the fate of first nature is always at any moment being decided. New technical developments, such as GM, are always significant and arresting because of the way we discern in them the irreversibility of our economic and political decisions and practices. To commit to GM, for example, is to know that the pre-GM moment will not come again and that it will create a certain fatedness, becoming part of "second nature." But at the same time, we also know that there is nothing fated about the commitment itself.

In the end, though, suggestive as some of these Adornian arguments are, I do not think they, or any other arguments I have discussed here, finally resolve the aporia of the demarcation between natural and unnatural. Susan Buck-Morss wrote in her discussion of Adorno's negative dialectics that "where nature confronted men as a mythic power Adorno called for the control of that nature by reason; but where rational control of nature took the form of domination, Adorno exposed such instrumental reason as a new mythology" (1977, p. 58). While this may be true, the key issue remains as to how we decide what constitutes a "rational" control of nature, what exactly counts as its domination, and why.

None of this, however, means, as I have argued elsewhere (Soper, 1996, pp. 33–34), that we can do whatever we choose to the environment or ourselves and still expect the planet and its various life-forms, including our own, to survive and flourish. We persist, then, in certain forms of biotechnological intervention very much at our own peril. Habermas noted in this connection the "symptomatic revulsion" we feel at the breaching of the species barrier that we had naively assumed to be inviolable—an "ethical virgin soil," as he puts it, quoting Otfried Hoffe (Habermas, 2002, pp. 39–40). He also argues against genetic programming, observing that "many of us seem to have the intuition that we should not weigh human life, not even in its earliest stages, either against the freedom (and competitiveness) of research, or against the concern with safeguarding an industrial edge, or against the wish for a healthy child, or even against the prospect (assumed *arguendo*) of new treatments for severe genetic diseases" (p. 68). And he rightly spoke of a Rubicon that we should be wary of crossing. It may indeed be difficult finally to justify such forms of "revulsion," but that is no reason to disregard them. There are, after all, aspects of human existence and response we may do better to acknowledge rather than seek to rationalize.[6] Even if we cannot point to any essential or universal aspects of ourselves that underlie our forms of resistance to specific forms of biotechnology, such intuitions are always to be attended to as signaling, not so much the limits of what we *can* do to ourselves and other creatures and the rest of nature, but what we can do and *still expect to live well,* to be happy, and to experience the rewards of membership of an ethical community. It is, in other words, one thing to recognize the relative autonomy of our political powers respecting the use of nature and our technical capacities to act on them, but it is another to suppose we could ever escape the constraints our nature imposes on what we can enjoy or experience as practically feasible or morally acceptable. If, then, the request to respect nature is construed in these terms, then it seems perfectly valid; indeed without it, it would seem impossible even to begin to make the distinctions between human nature and the nature destroyed by human culture, or between ecological and ideological conceptions of nature, which are so important to disentangling the oppositions of contemporary theory around the idea of "nature."

ACKNOWLEDGMENT

An earlier version of this chapter appeared under the title "Unnatural Times? The Social Imaginary and the Future of Nature" in *Nature, Society and Environmental Crisis*, ed. Bob Carter and Nickie Charles (Malden, Mass.: Wiley-Blackwell, 2010), 222–35.

NOTES

1. Cf. Dollimore (1991, pp. 64–74, 225–26, 233–34). For Foucault's account of the "reverse discourse," whereby those labeled "perverse" employ the same vocabulary and categories of the "natural" to assert their legitimacy as those who have disqualified them, see Foucault (1980, pp. 101–2).

2. Kaebnick cites, among others, Hallman et al. (2004); Marris et al. (2002); and Sosin and Richards (2005).

3. Cf. the argument to this effect developed in Kaebnick (2007); see also Kaebnick (2008).

4. Haraway's cyborg manifesto has inspired numerous commentaries and articles. For an extensive selection, see Gray (1995). For some more skeptical and polemical responses, see Bordo (1990); Soper (1999); McCormick (2002).

5. OncoMouse was developed by DuPont for the study of breast cancer. See Haraway (1997).

6. Although developed primarily in response to philosophical skepticism on "other minds," aspects of Stanley Cavell's argument around the idea of "acknowledgment" in part 4 of *The Claim of Reason* (1979) have some relevance in this context.

REFERENCES

Adorno, T. 1973. *History and Freedom: Lectures, 1964–1965.* Ed. R. Tiedemann. London: Wiley.
———. 1997. *Aesthetic Theory.* Ed. G. Adorno and R. Tiedemann. Trans. R. Hullot-Kentor. London: Athlone.
———. 2006. *Negative Dialectics.* Trans. E. B. Ashton. London: Routledge.
Benton, T. 1989. "Marxism and Natural Limits." *New Left Review* 178 (November–December): 51–86. Reprinted in P. Osborne, ed., *Socialism and the Limits of Liberalism*, pp. 241–69, London: Verso, 1990.
———. 1992. "Ecology, Socialism and the Mastery of Nature: A Reply to Reiner Grundmann." *New Left Review* 194 (July–August): 55–74.
Bordo, S. 1990. "Feminism, Postmodernism, and Gender-Skepticism." In *Feminism/Postmodernism*, ed. L. Nicholson, pp. 133–56. London: Routledge.
Buck-Morss, S. 1977. *The Origin of Negative Dialectics.* London: Macmillan.
Butler, J. 1990. *Gender Trouble: Feminism and the Subversion of Identity.* London: Routledge.
———. 1993. *Bodies That Matter.* London: Routledge.
Cavell, S. 1979. *The Claim of Reason: Wittgenstein, Skepticism, Morality, and Tragedy.* Oxford: Clarendon.

Dollimore, J. 1991. *Sexual Dissidence: Augustine to Wilde, Freud to Foucault.* Oxford: Clarendon.

Foucault, M. 1980. *History of Sexuality.* Vol. 1, *An Introduction.* New York: Vintage.

Freud, S. 1974–86. *The Pelican Freud Library.* 15 vols. Ed. A. Richards. Harmondsworth, U.K.: Penguin.

Gray, C. H., ed. 1995. *The Cyborg Handbook.* London: Routledge.

Habermas, J. 2002. *The Future of Human Nature.* Cambridge, U.K.: Polity.

Hallman, W. K., et al. 2004. "Americans and GM Food: Knowledge, Opinion, and Interest in 2004." Publication no. RR-1104-007. New Brunswick, N.J.: Food Policy Institute, Cook College, Rutgers University. www.foodpolicyinstitute.org/docs/reports/NationalStudy2004.pdf.

Haraway, D. 1991. *Simians, Cyborgs, and Women: The Reinvention of Nature.* London: Free Association.

———. 1997. *ModestWitness@Second Millennium: FemaleMan© Meets OncoMouse™.* London: Routledge.

Hardt, M., and A. Negri. 2000. *Empire.* Cambridge, Mass.: Harvard University Press.

Jeffreys, S. 1990. *Anticlimax.* London: Women's Press.

Kaebnick, G. E. 2007. "Putting Concerns about Nature in Context: The Case of Agricultural Biotechnology." *Perspectives in Biology and Medicine* 50 (4): 572–84.

———. 2008. "Reasons of the Heart: Emotions, Rationality, and the 'Wisdom of Repugnance.'" *Hastings Center Report* 38 (4): 36–45.

Kant, I. 1987. *Critique of Judgment.* Ed. W. S. Pluhar. London: Hackett.

Marris, C., et al. 2002. "Public Perceptions of Agricultural Biotechnologies in Europe: Final Report of the PABE Research Project." Commission of European Communities. Available at http://csec.lancs.ac.uk/archive/pabe/docs/pabe_finalreport.pdf.

McCormick, B. 2002. "The Island of Dr. Haraway." *Environmental Ethics* 22 (Winter): 409–18.

Nuffield Council on Bioethics. 1999. "Genetically Modified Crops: The Ethical and Social Issues." London.

Rich, A. 1983. "Compulsory Heterosexuality and Lesbian Existence." In *The Signs Reader,* ed. E. and E. K. Abel, pp. 139–68. Chicago: University of Chicago Press.

Silverman, K. 1988. "Masochism and Male Subjectivity." *Camera Obscura* (17 May): 31–66.

Soper, K. 1995. *What Is Nature? Culture, Politics, and the Non-Human.* Oxford: Blackwell.

———. 1996. "Nature/'Nature.'" In *FutureNatural,* ed. G. Robertson et al., pp. 22–34. London: Routledge.

———. 1999. "Of OncoMice and FemaleMen: Donna Haraway on Cyborg Ontology." *Women: A Cultural Review* 10 (2): 167–72.

Sosin, J., and M. D. Richards. 2005. "What Will Consumers Do? Understanding Consumer Response When Meat and Milk from Cloned Animals Reach Supermarkets." Washington, D.C.: KRC Research.

Streiffer, R. 2003. "In Defense of the Moral Relevance of Species Boundaries." *American Journal of Bioethics* 3 (3): 37–38.

Vogel, S. 2006. "Why 'Nature' Has No Place in Environmental Philosophy." Presentation at the Hastings Center, Garrison, N.Y., November 9.

CHAPTER TWO

In Defense of Living Nature

Finding Common Ground in a Medieval Tradition

Jean Porter, Ph.D.

Science and traditional Christianity have often been regarded as adversaries between whom there can be, at best, a mutual pact of silence and disengagement. Yet the current environmental crisis has prompted thoughtful men and women in both camps to reconsider the terms of this standoff and to ask whether it might be possible to find, at the very least, common ground for shared action on behalf of urgently needed reforms. Among committed Christians, we are beginning to see a growing dismay over the ways their cherished beliefs have been co-opted by a reactionary and plutocratic political regime. Men and women of science, for their part, have understandably been reluctant to enter into conversation with theologians and church leaders who all too often reject out of hand the very premises of their life's work. Yet they too have begun asking whether they are closing themselves off from powerful allies with whom they might share common sensibilities of appreciation for the natural world and a shared commitment to respect and preserve it in its beauty and integrity. As E. O. Wilson put it in *Creation: An Appeal to Save Life on Earth,* addressed to an anonymous Baptist pastor, "I suggest that we set aside our differences in order to save the Creation. The defense of living Nature is a universal value" (2007, p. 4).

For the past several years, my own work has focused on the early scholastic conception of a natural law and its contemporary relevance.[1] This research has convinced me that there is indeed a basis for cooperation between scientists and religious believers, grounded in mutual sensibilities and perhaps, for at least some scientists and some believers, in shared beliefs about the integrity and value of the natural order. What I have in mind is, not so much the scholastics' theory of the natural law per se, but the assumptions and the general theological approach that undergirded it. The scholastic concept of the natural law could only have emerged within a context that was friendly to the idea of nature and optimistic about the capacities of the human intellect to understand and appropriately value the natural world—even apart from the guidance of revelation and Christian belief. This context, in turn, reflected a robust philosophy of nature that began to emerge in the late eleventh century and, correlatively, a broadly expansive and open theology that emphasized the intrinsic intelligibility and goodness of the created order. Here we find starting points for real common ground between religion and science, or at least between some important constituencies in each camp. It may seem odd, or even perverse, to turn to the early medieval period as a resource for addressing a postmodern problem, yet this approach offers at least one advantage in that it enables us to bypass the distinctively modern congeries of assumptions and commitments that lead us to assume that scientific and religious worldviews must necessarily be at odds.

The Scholastic Conception of Nature

The story I want to tell begins in the prescholastic period, in the centers of learning associated with the great European cathedrals, where distinguished scholars laid the foundations for a systematic philosophy of nature. They are characterized, first of all, by their commitment to Platonic philosophy, particularly as it was mediated to them through Plato's *Timaeus* (the only Platonic dialogue available in Latin translation at this time) and a number of Platonically minded theologians from earlier eras. As Winthrop Wetherbee says, for these scholars "to study nature was in effect to decode the *Timaeus*" (1988, p. 34), and they were particularly concerned with reconciling Plato's account of the fabrication of the world in that dialogue with the creation story given in Genesis. Their devotion to Plato and his commentators generated views that seem strange to us, including (for some) a belief in a world-soul that exists apart from both God and the visible universe and a tendency to personify Nature, speaking as if she were an entity in her own right.

Nonetheless, these odd views should not blind us to the importance of their work; it marks the first moment when Christian scholars made a systematic attempt to reconcile Scripture with philosophical accounts of the origins and intrinsic character of the visible world. By no means did they proceed by imposing a simple scriptural narrative onto the philosophy, as if the latter had nothing distinctive to contribute to our understanding of the world—or, indeed, to the interpretation of Scripture itself. Given the current state of our own impasse between scriptural and scientific approaches to questions of origins, it is startling to read William of Conches coolly announcing in *Glosae super Platonem* that the Genesis story of the creation of Adam and Eve "must not be believed literally" (Gregory, 1988, p. 65). More generally, these scholars insisted on the intelligibility of natural processes, which should be understood in terms of the unfolding of intrinsic principles through natural causes. They did not deny the doctrine of the creation, but they insisted that God created the world as an integral whole, with internal principles of action sufficient to generate the processes of growth and decay that sustain the created order. Hence, they emphasized God's creative wisdom while de-emphasizing the role played by miraculous interventions into the cosmic order.

By the middle of the twelfth century, the Neoplatonic natural philosophy developed by the scholars of Chartres and their pupils began to be supplanted by the philosophical works of Aristotle and his Greek and Arabic commentators, which were increasingly being made available in Latin translations. By this point the scholastic period was well established, with the university system, centered on a stable community of scholars and students pursuing a set curriculum of study, beginning to dominate professional training, as well as intellectual life. The natural philosophy of the early twelfth century played a central role in this system, if only because it was a standard part of the so-called arts curriculum, the basic course of studies required of nearly every university student. This was doubly significant. Because natural philosophy was a part of the arts curriculum, its scholars demanded and won independence for it as a discipline, as part of their efforts to secure their independence as a faculty. At the same time, every scholar in the medieval university had to receive a degree from the faculty of arts in order to pass on to further studies, and this meant that not only philosophers but also every theologian and lawyer would be trained in natural philosophy.

By this time, the natural philosophy in question was predominantly Aristotelian rather than Platonic, thanks in part to the fact that Aristotle's treatises, together with their Muslim commentaries, served as the foundation of the arts curriculum. It would take us beyond the scope of this chapter to examine the details of this worldview, but certain points should be noted. The proponents of Aristotelian natural philosophy typically understood "nature" in terms of the nature of particular creatures, that is to say, as the complex of intrinsic principles expressed in the mode of activity proper to a creature of a given kind. This interpretation set them apart from their Platonically minded predecessors, who were more inclined to speak of nature as an autonomous generative and directive force that could direct or instruct individual creatures from without. For this reason, many of the characteristic motifs of twelfth-century natural philosophy, including the idea of a world soul and the image of Nature as a personified being, more or less disappear in this period. Thirteenth-century thinkers sometimes spoke of nature as the whole complex of existing beings, but they tended to identify nature so understood with creation, that is, as the term of God's creative activity. At the same time, thirteenth-century natural philosophy preserved much of the spirit of its twelfth-century antecedents. If scholars in this period were more hesitant than their predecessors to speak of nature as an autonomous principle of action, they nonetheless affirmed its relative independence. They continued to look for explanations of natural phenomena in terms of intrinsic principles rather than appealing to God's inscrutable will or focusing on possible symbolic or allegorical interpretations. Correlatively, they insisted on the intelligibility and goodness of natural phenomena, seen on their own terms and as expressions of the wisdom and love of God as creator.

Science and Christianity

What does any of this have to offer to contemporary efforts to find common ground between scientists and traditional Christians? First, and most obviously, the scholastic construal of nature as a system of intelligible causes, more or less autonomous in its operations and comprehensible on its own terms, suggests an analogy with the scientist's commitment to give an independently verifiable account of natural processes.[2] I do not want to press the analogy too far—medieval philosophy of nature is profoundly different, in both its aims and its methodologies, from the intellectual commitments and practices undergirding contemporary scientific inquiry. Yet these two ways of accounting for the natural world do at least share a relative optimism about human capacities to understand the fundamental principles or laws governing the world on their own terms, apart from any kind of special revelation. By the same token, scholastic theology, developed as it is within the parameters of this natural philosophy, provides us with an example of a theological trajectory that is not fundamentally hostile to independent inquiry into the origins and causal principles of the natural world.

This brings me to what is potentially a second meeting point between scientists and Christian believers. For the scholastics, the intelligibility of natural processes in terms of intrinsic causal principles was invariably correlated with some idea of natural goodness. They were well aware of the ambiguities and dangers of naturalness taken as a normative standard, but they nonetheless held on to the fundamental claim that nature, realized fully and without distortion, is good, and good in terms that are intrinsic to natural processes themselves—that is to say, not instrumentally, by reference to extrinsic desires and needs. This was so, whether nature was understood in terms of an all-embracing cosmic order or by reference to the distinctive natures of specific kinds of creatures. The world with its order and regularity taken as a whole was perceived as beautiful in itself, an appropriate reflection of divine simplicity and order at the level of finite, mutable existence. The goodness intrinsic to distinctive natures was understood, more or less following Aristotle, in terms of the ideal of perfection, that is to say, full development and activity in accordance with intrinsic principles of operation. Thus understood, the beauty and goodness that we intuitively perceive in the natural world reflect a substantive ideal of flourishing that represents the necessary correlate to the intelligibility of natural kinds.

Understood from either religious or scientific perspective, the scholastic commitment to the intrinsic goodness of nature clearly has much to offer to collaborative efforts in defense of the environment (Wilson, 2007, p. 5). It suggests a framework within which to affirm that nonhuman nature, however we understand it, has a value that cannot simply be reduced to its instrumental usefulness but, on the contrary, claims our respect and forbearance. Wilson remarks at one point that "we can agree that each species, however inconspicuous and humble it may seem to be to us at this moment, is a masterpiece of biology and well worth saving" (p. 5). This reflects a widely held sense that natural entities and processes are intrinsically good—a sentiment all the more striking because it is so frequently voiced by those whose scientific or philosophical, or indeed theological, positions should rule it out. Of course, we cannot just assume that these kinds of remarks reflect a deep apprehension of the natural and metaphysical principles structuring the world and our perceptions of it. I happen to believe that myself, but I am well aware that claims about natural goodness must be formulated carefully and defended against formidable philosophical objections. I would only suggest that just as we cannot embrace the scholastic commitment to the goodness of nature without qualification, neither should we dismiss it out of hand. This perspective does challenge some of our most entrenched philosophical assumptions, yet for that very reason it is worth reconsidering in this context. After all, there is a case to be made that our pervasive assumption that nature has no normative significance or value, except insofar as we make something of it, goes a long way toward explaining how we have arrived at the present point of crisis.

Of course, any history of attitudes toward the environment will also need to take account of the long-standing Christian commitment to affirming human dominion over nature, with its correlative claim that nonhuman entities were created and continue to exist for the sake of human welfare. It is difficult to reconcile this perspective with the warm, sometimes ecstatic affirmations of the integrity and goodness of the created world considered on its own terms—in fact, we shouldn't try too hard to reconcile the two. They represent an ongoing tension within the Christian tradition itself, a tension that invites reflective analysis and (hopefully) a reasoned resolution, a task made all the more urgent by the environmental crisis we face.

Once again, the scholastics offer resources for thinking through the relevant issues, even though they do not develop the specific line of argument I now want to sketch. What is at stake in the Christian emphasis on dominion is after all a particular reading of Scripture, which takes God's command to our first parents recorded in Genesis 1:28 to fill the Earth and to exercise dominion over it as being the final and definitive word on the proper human relationship to nonhuman creation.[3] But, as I have already suggested, the scholastics are not nearly so bound to literalist or fundamentalist readings of Scripture as we might assume. For one thing, they understood the authority of Scripture in such a way as to place decisive interpretative weight on the canon taken as a whole, rather than focusing on individual texts in the current fundamentalist fashion. Moreover, they had learned from their patristic forbears that Scripture must be interpreted with attentiveness to context and genre if we are to apprehend the true intention of its author—God, ultimately, but also the human authors through whom God speaks. Most importantly, at least from our standpoint, they interpreted Scripture within a context of wider assumptions, aims, and ideals described by eminent historian Richard Southern as "scholastic humanism." As he explains:

It was the twelfth century innovators who first introduced systematic order into the mass of intellectual material which they had inherited in a largely uncoordinated form from the ancient world. The general aim of their work was to produce a complete and systematic body of knowledge, clarified by the refinements of criticism, and presented as the consensus of competent judges. Doctrinally the method for achieving this consensus was a progression from commentary to questioning, and from questioning to systematization. . . . In principle, they aimed at restoring to fallen mankind, so far as was possible, that perfect system of knowledge which had been in the possession or within the reach of mankind at the moment of creation. (1995, pp. 4–5)[4]

The "orthodox Christian view of the world" at which the scholastics aimed was thus nothing less than a theory of everything, in which all that is humanly knowable is in fact known and, what is more, properly understood. This ideal is reminiscent of contemporary aspirations within the domain of physics to arrive at a unified scientific theory. Again, I would not want to push this comparison too far, but it does suggest that the scholastics would have shared with us an ideal of reason as a comprehensive and unifying principle of knowledge. They were not hostile to reason, nor did they reject the philosopher's ideal of a cogent system developed out of rational inquiry. We might say they wanted to beat non-Christian philosophers at their own game, deploying the techniques of rational analysis in order to offer a better, more comprehensive system of thought than the philosophers could hope to provide.

This ideal governed the scholastic reading of texts—not only Scripture but an array of other texts of Jewish, Islamic, and classical, as well as Christian, provenance, which were regarded as having lesser but still weighty authority. The lesser texts preserved fragments of the truth while Scripture provided the interpretative key for reuniting these fragments into a systematic and comprehensible whole. Scripture would illuminate and confirm the insights established independently of revelation, rather than substituting for them or simply overruling seeming inconsistencies. Practically speaking, this meant that for the scholastics, theology as a discipline was answerable, to some extent at least, to the best insights of these non-Christian traditions of rational inquiry. Taken in the context of current dialogues, this ideal would imply that we Christians cannot simply dismiss or ignore inconvenient philosophical or scientific or cultural perspectives in the name of the supposed supremacy and self-sufficiency of faith. Rather, we must offer the most comprehensive and widely persuasive accounts of the world as seen from the perspective of faith that we can manage, ones in which our interlocutors can recognize and embrace their own best insights.

All Things Seen and Unseen

That is all very well, you might say, but how does this help address the scriptural texts that seem to affirm a one-sided human dominion over nature? My specific point is that the scholastic project of interpreting Scripture in continuity, as far as possible, with non-Christian perspectives provided, and indeed required, considerable flexibility in construing the scriptural texts themselves. The scholastics aimed at a synthetic reading of a complex and diverse canon, developed within parameters set by a wider synthesis of philosophical considerations to which they were, at least implicitly, accountable. If they were to develop the needed synthesis, they could not allow any one text to carry definitive and interpretative weight; rather, they had to construct narratives that tied together diverse scriptural and (we might say) secular perspectives in cogent and illuminating ways. The story of human dominion over nature exemplifies one such narrative, but Scripture also contains the resources for a counternarrative, one that gives priority to the autonomy of the nonhuman natural order, its value, and its independent transparency to God's creative and providential care.

I have already noted that the scholastics placed a great deal of weight on the independent goodness of nature considered as a set of intrinsic principles of operation. The specific terms in which they formulated this insight were philosophical, but their motives for insisting on it were theological—drawn in part from opposition to contemporaneous heterodox views according to which matter and the visible world are necessarily deformed or evil, but drawn even more so from the affirmations of the goodness of the natural world that we find beginning in the creation narratives themselves and that continue throughout the canon as a whole. At some points the Hebrew Scriptures emphasize not only the independence but the otherness of nonhuman nature and its indifference to human concerns—as Job is forcefully reminded, only God knows when the mountain goat gives birth; only God has freed the wild ass, yoked the wild ox, and tamed Leviathan, playing with it as a pet bird (Job. 9:1–18, 41:1–11). We can well imagine a scriptural narrative informed by these considerations and focused on these and similar texts from the wisdom literature and Psalms, as well as Job—one in which God's overarching purposes include the whole array of created reality, all things "seen and unseen" as the creeds put it, functioning together to glorify the Creator in their independence from human purposes and designs. In this view, "dominion" would be nothing more (or less!) than the privilege of participating in, fostering, and safeguarding the independence and operations of natural processes, enjoyed by men and women because we are capable of grasping and appreciating what these mean, and what their true value is. This privilege emphatically would not be understood as a license to usurp God's ultimate authority over creation, or much less as a mandate to despoil and distort the nonhuman world in pursuit of our own aims.

The narrative I have just sketched does in fact find echoes in scholastic Christian theology, more than I can trace at this point. Why have we been so slow to make it explicit? The first thing to be said is that we—I now mean we Christians— have begun to do so, although not necessarily in these specific terms. Even so, the twentieth and early-twenty-first centuries do seem late for developing this kind of narrative. But then, explicit attentiveness to environmental concerns does not go back much earlier than this era. This is not surprising when we consider that we have only recently begun to understand that human action can have a direct and permanent impact on natural processes. We have only recently begun to perceive the world in terms of ecosystems and biological (in contrast to metaphysical or conceptual) species, entities of a sort that comprise objects of human action, for better or worse—so far, unfortunately, mostly for the worst.

But we are now well and truly fallen from the Eden of innocence with respect to our own destructive powers vis-à-vis the natural, living world we inhabit. Instead of dominion, we find ourselves compelled to "the defense of living nature"—a challenge that does not admit easy or complete execution, but one we must take up nonetheless. We can meet this challenge effectively only through large-scale, collective action, with the aim of transforming our overarching systems of consumption and exchange in such a way as to minimize their environmental impact and, so far as possible, to reverse the damage that has already been done. This kind of large-scale action raises considerations, and calls for a kind of systems-oriented thinking, that take it beyond the immediate scope of scholastic natural law theory. Indeed, we are at this point at the limits of nearly every moral theory, whether philosophical or theological, because with a few, largely unpersuasive exceptions, these theories take individual human actions to be the proper starting points and focus for normative analysis.[5] Indeed, there are good philosophical reasons for thinking that this approach is both appropriate and inevitable, and recent work in cognitive theory and comparative psychology lends credence to this view.[6] Nonetheless, so long as we stay focused at the level of the discrete actions of individual men and women, we will only get so far in our attempts to develop a workable environmental ethic. For one thing, under normal circumstances, individual acts, taken in themselves, have at most a negligible effect on the environment. Their impact depends on their place in a large-scale system of causal interactions, which is why systems and forms of life, rather than individual acts, would seem the proper focus for an environmental ethic. What is more, our judgments and sensibilities as agents are invariably shaped by our perceptions of ourselves as operating within a delimited range—men and women whose powers to respond to others and to bring about changes, while real and important, are limited. It is not clear that we should even want to change this aspect of ourselves—we would not want to focus exclusively on our responsibilities to the natural order, at the expense of neglecting the claims and needs of other individuals.

Yet these difficulties, while distinctive and uniquely problematic in an environmental context, are not altogether unprecedented. In the modern period, we see similar difficulties arising within economic contexts, in which large-scale market forces, rather than individual acts, normally determine whatever good or bad effects flow from our collective attempts to make money and to spend it. The scholastics began to identify similar difficulties in their analysis of the institution of property, which they regarded as closely correlated (in its present forms) with structures of dominion and servitude. These analogies reinforce the point that environmental ethics is properly focused in the first instance on the appropriate design of systems rather than on individual actions, yet they also serve to remind us that individual actions can and do have an impact, most immediately and directly in the political realm. After all, the systems in question are products of collective human action and (to some degree) conscious design, and they can be modified, perhaps drastically, through concerted collective action. It seems to me that what we lack, at least in the context of environmental ethics, is not so much knowledge of what kinds of changes we need to make but the political will to demand these changes and the courage to carry them out and sustain them. It is at this point that a renewed sensibility, shaped by a deeper appreciation of the value and integrity—and, perhaps, the divine origins—of living nature can have its most immediate and far-reaching impact.

NOTES

1. I bring together and reflect on the significance of my work in this period in *Natural and Divine Law: Reclaiming the Tradition for Christian Ethics* (1999) and *Nature as Reason: A Thomistic Theory of the Natural Law* (2005). Throughout this chapter, I draw on the arguments presented in these books, and further arguments and documentation may be found there. See, in particular, *Natural and Divine Law,*

pp. 34–62, on the social and intellectual context of scholastic natural philosophy, and pp. 63–120, on the scholastic philosophy of nature and its continued viability; see also *Nature as Reason,* pp. 82–140, for a further defense of an Aristotelian teleology in the light of contemporary biology and philosophy and science.

2. In reaction to earlier (and still widely prevalent) views, several historians have recently argued that at least some key elements of contemporary ideals of scientific inquiry are in continuity with, and even dependent on, classical and medieval philosophies of nature; two notable examples would be Grant (1996) and Lindberg (2008).

3. For an extensive and illuminating discussion of medieval Christian interpretations of this text, see Cohen (1989, pp. 221–70).

4. He goes on to offer an illuminating analysis of the way this ideal shaped the scholastic approach to scriptural interpretation at pp. 102–33.

5. I don't regard virtue- or character-based theories of ethics as exceptions to this rule because they also take individual acts as a necessary starting point and focus for normative reflection, insofar as these reflect (and perhaps also foster) the development of one's virtue and character. However, a number of philosophers and some theologians have defended the radical consequentialist view that individual human acts as such carry no special normative significance, the upshot being that we are equally responsible for every consequence of every act and every omission. The locus classicus for this approach is Singer (1972); see also Singer (1994). Other influential examples include Parfit (1984); Kagan (1989); and (among theologians) Hallett (1995). Bennett (1995) defends a similar claim, but with important reservations on analytic grounds.

6. I make the case for the former claim in *Nature as Reason* (Porter, 2005, pp. 288–308). Marc Hauser, who specializes in comparative cognitive psychology, marshaled an impressive body of evidence, including data taken from his own research, to make the case that our tendency to focus on human acts, and to distinguish different causal pathways within action, is "hard-wired," even though the specific normative valence we give these distinctions is, by and large, culturally determined (2006).

REFERENCES

Bennett, J. 1995. *The Act Itself.* Oxford: Oxford University Press.
Cohen, J. 1989. *"Be Fertile and Increase, Fill the Earth and Master It": The Ancient and Medieval Career of a Biblical Text.* Ithaca, N.Y.: Cornell University Press.
Grant, E. 1996. *The Foundations of Modern Science in the Middle Ages: Their Religious, Institutional, and Intellectual Contexts.* Cambridge, U.K.: Cambridge University Press.
Gregory, T. 1988. "The Platonic Inheritance." In *A History of Twelfth Century Philosophy,* ed. P. Dronke, pp. 54–80. Cambridge, U.K.: Cambridge University Press.
Hallett, G. L. 1995. *Greater Good: The Case for Proportionalism.* Washington, D.C.: Georgetown University Press.
Hauser, M. 2006. *Moral Minds: How Nature Designed Our Universal Sense of Right and Wrong.* New York: HarperCollins.
Kagan, S. 1989. *The Limits of Morality.* Oxford: Oxford University Press.

Lindberg, D. C. 2008. *The Beginnings of Western Science: The European Scientific Tradition in Philosophical, Religious, and Institutional Context, 600 B.C. to A.D. 1450.* Rev. ed. Chicago: University of Chicago Press.

Parfit, D. 1984. *Reasons and Persons.* Oxford: Oxford University Press.

Porter, J. 1999. *Natural and Divine Law: Reclaiming the Tradition for Christian Ethics.* Grand Rapids, Mich.: Eerdmans.

———. 2005. *Nature as Reason: A Thomistic Theory of the Natural Law.* Grand Rapids, Mich.: Eerdmans.

Singer, P. 1972. "Famine, Affluence, and Morality." *Philosophy and Public Affairs* 1:229–43.

———. 1994. *Rethinking Life and Death: The Collapse of Our Traditional Ethics.* New York: St. Martin's.

Southern, R. W. 1995. *Scholastic Humanism and the Unification of Europe.* Vol. 1, *Foundations.* Oxford: Blackwell.

Wetherbee, W. 1988. "Philosophy, Cosmology, and the Twelfth-Century Renaissance." In *A History of Twelfth-Century Philosophy,* ed. P. Dronke, pp. 21–53. Cambridge, U.K.: Cambridge University Press.

Wilson, E. O. 2007. *The Creation: An Appeal to Save Life on Earth.* New York: Norton.

CHAPTER THREE

Nature as Absence

The Logic of Nature and Culture in Social Contract Theory

Bruce Jennings, M.A.

Does the concept of nature have any force or function in ethics? Strong theorists today generally answer "no." Judith Butler and John Rawls, while they may agree on little else, both dispense with nature as a normative category. When the category of the natural appears in the humanities today (at least where postmodernism or social constructivism hold sway), it is usually seen as a component of the "rhetoric of reaction," and it seems to operate under the sign of cultural imperialism and ideological domination (Hirschman, 1991). Philosophically, the concept of the normatively natural and the concept of human nature seem to entail an outmoded ethnocentric and antihistorical essentialism. Nature is an ideological category used to impose rules and values on a society or on certain marginalized groups within society.

This was not always so. In this chapter I explore and seek to recover a mode of discourse in which the concept of nature or the natural is substantive and central yet avoids the philosophical pitfall of reactionary essentialism in which it is no longer plausible (or possible) to believe. I find the mode of discourse I seek in early-modern social contract theory, especially the versions of that theory developed by Thomas Hobbes and Jean-Jacques Rousseau.

I approach this analysis more in the fashion of a literary critic and a historian of ideas than as a moral or environmental philosopher. I do not seek in these texts a theory to defend. I aim instead to understand how important concepts and categories take on their meaning within larger conceptual and philosophical frameworks. I am interested especially in how such frameworks both enable and impede the expression of certain insights and understandings. All theorists, like all speakers of natural language, must employ conceptual frameworks that are available to them in their historical context (Pocock, 1973). Like poets, strong theorists may exercise unusual creativity in how they shape and deploy these conceptual frameworks, but they are not free to invent a whole new language for expressing original ideas. The thinkers I find most interesting struggle with their inherited and available discourses and conceptual frameworks, pushing concepts to, and a little past, the limits of their conventional meanings, finding ambivalence where only valence had been seen before. Social contract theory as a genre of discourse is one such enabling and constraining framework, and Hobbes and Rousseau are strong theorists who strive to say more than can be said within it. The drama of their thought—if not all the lines of its script—should once more become the drama of our own.

I also turn to study the conceptual structure of early social contract theory because in it one finds a rich, complex, and nuanced understanding of three master categories of modern thought, if not of Western thought as a whole: nature, culture, and humanity or humanness. Hobbes and Rousseau did not consider nature to be the foundation or the limiting essence determining the content of morality. They did not see culture as a veneer overlaying nature, nor did they see nature as a mere figment of cultural imagination, a construct. Like Wittgensteinian philosophical therapists, avant la lettre, they set those unprofitable questions aside in favor of a different way of thinking. They changed the subject.

The new question is: How do the natural and the cultural interpenetrate and combine to produce the human? Nature alone cannot realize humanity. The divine is no longer on stage, nor is it part of the story the early contractarians tell. Culture brings forth humanity—by which I mean human self-realization and the human good—on both the individual and the communal level. But culture can do this only by reaching into and drawing on nature. Culture can also deform and corrupt; it can actualize the human stain as well as the human good. In either case, culture is in concert with nature to produce some form of humanity. An important passage from *On the Social Contract* adumbrates the possibilities of a perspective that moves away from natural or ontological essentialism, although we must bear in mind that it is only one of several formulations Rousseau offers on this recurring theme—indeed, the master theme—of his work. "The passage from the state of nature to the civil state produces a remarkable change in man," Rousseau writes, "by substituting justice for instinct in his behavior and giving his actions the morality they previously lacked. . . . Although in this state he deprives himself of several advantages given him by nature, he gains such great ones, . . . that if the abuses of this new condition did not often degrade him beneath the condition he left, he ought ceaselessly to bless the happy moment that tore him away from it forever, and that changed him from a stupid, limited animal into an intelligent being and a man" (Rousseau, 1978, pp. 55–56).

Goodness and justice are culturally natural—nature's potential realized through culture. Yet evil and injustice are also "natural" in their potential and cultural in their realization, their embodiment in social action, and their embeddedness in historical time. Morally and politically Janus-faced, nature can be well realized through culture into virtuous, communal human life, or it can be deformed through culture into vicious, deracinated human life.

Why not simply say that nature is value-neutral and that both good and evil, justice and injustice, virtue and vice come from culture? Because the concept of culture alone cannot bear that philosophical or anthropological burden. Only operating in an interplay with the concept of the natural do the form giving, rule governed, meaning making capacities of culture become sources of normative force and interpretive understanding.

Three Snapshots of Social Contract Theory

Before proceeding further with the discussion, for those readers without a recent acquaintance with the texts of Hobbes, Locke, and Rousseau, a brief synopsis of their social contract theories may be helpful.

Thomas Hobbes (1588–1679)

Hobbes supported the monarchy of Charles I against the Puritan revolution during the 1640s. When the English Civil War broke out pitting the Royalists against the supporters of Parliament, who eventually prevailed (King Charles I was defeated, tried, and executed in 1649), many in the king's court went into exile in France, where Hobbes also fled in 1640. He became associated with the Royalists, and they promoted his work. After the publication of *Leviathan* in 1651, however, he fell out of favor with the court in exile and had to return to England later that year, ironically, under the protection of the Parliamentarian government. In his various political and psychological writings, Hobbes presented several versions of his account of the state of nature, the founding social contract, and the nature and justification for sovereign authority established by that collective agreement. The last and definitive version of his theory is found in his masterpiece, *Leviathan*.

He tried to develop his political and ethical theory in quasi-geometric fashion, beginning from premises and propositions about human nature and psychology and drawing conclusions concerning politics and obligation. Human psychology for Hobbes was pain-avoiding and pleasure-seeking; human behavior—whether natural or cultural—was driven by the passions, not by reason. No ideas or moral virtues were innate. The main "natural" psychological motivation was fear, especially fear of violent death. For Hobbes the state of nature was also a state of potential and actual perpetual conflict, a war of all against all. It was a condition before the invention of morality, with only one principle of natural right: self-preservation. That gave each individual unlimited freedom and license to do anything necessary to protect himself, including engaging in preemptive first strikes. Hobbes did not posit that humans were naturally aggressive, cruel, or prone to violence. On the contrary, he thought that these behaviors were artificially constructed and that people were miserable in this condition. The state of nature/war was the result of insecurity, the lack of a creditable deterrent, the lack of authoritative common rules for mutual cooperation and living, and the lack of a common power to enforce those rules. In a word, the lack of a sovereign authority.

The social contract is the vehicle for creating that common sovereignty via consent of the subjects. Once established, the reasonable and legitimate authority of the sovereign is unified and absolute. Hobbes rejected the notion of constitutional government or separation of powers. There is no moral limit on the sovereign's laws. There is, however, one natural limit, and that is the right of self-preservation. If the sovereign threatens a subject's life, then the two revert to a state of nature vis-à-vis one another. The civic bond is broken, and with it all obligation, not so much because a higher natural right is invoked by the subject as because the sovereign's edict seriously threatening the life of the subject is a logical contradiction. It undermines the very grounds of sovereign authority, namely, protection and security of life. Survival of the strongest or most fortunate will be the amoral rule. Aside from capital punishment (and perhaps military conscription), however, the subject had no just cause for disobedience.

The Hobbesian sovereign defines the content of law and morality. He uses a notion of prepolitical "natural law," but it does not have the independent normative force for Hobbes that it did for Locke, and the last thing Hobbes wanted to do was set up a standard of transpolitical right that would justify (and motivate) disobedience or collective revolution. The positive laws of the sovereign need not be purely arbitrary, however. Strategic rationality and intelligence should guide the sovereign in promoting the commonwealth and in keeping the peace. Peace, tranquility, and order were the principal values in Hobbes's vision of civil society. Scientific knowledge should be promoted, but religious and metaphysical discourse should be curbed. Hobbes believed that it was religious extremism and the struggle to seize power under the guise of religious reform that led to the political turmoil in England during this period, and the state of nature is an analytic portrait of the social and political chaos of his time. Man without sovereign authority is too self-interested to cooperate effectively for there are no grounds for reasonable trust. Therefore, economic and technological progress suffers and man's material standard of living and his power over the exploitation of natural resources suffers.

John Locke (1632–1704)

During his lifetime, Hobbes had little direct influence on English politics. His defense of monarchy was not as reliable as the notion of tradition and the divine right of kings, defended by thinkers such as Hobbes's contemporary Robert Filmer. Indeed, social contract theory was one of the main discursive opponents of divine right theory in seventeenth-century England. Although Hobbes personally supported the Stuart monarchs, his theory did not necessary do so. Absolute sovereignty, not monarchy, is what his theory establishes. But that sovereignty could take the institutional form of an aristocracy or even a democracy. Because Rousseau also uses the social contract device to reach absolute sovereign authority, he seems to develop a democratic version of Hobbesian theory, albeit with an account of the state of nature that developmentally reaches a state of war, or something close to it, but not as a natural feature of the human condition.

Locke, who came about twenty to thirty years after Hobbes and sixty years before Rousseau, was active in the 1680s and 1690s. His version of contractarianism set out to refute Filmer and the divine right of kings (the first part of his main work of political theory, *Two Treatises of Government*) and to establish through moral consent a kind of sovereign authority that was not absolute (the second part of *Two Treatises of Government*). Locke wrote to defend the Glorious Revolution of 1688–89, not after the fact, as was long thought, but before the revolution that brought King William of Orange and Queen Mary to England and replaced the Stuart dynasty with the house of Hanover. (Locke's *Two Treatises of Government* was published anonymously and its dates of composition were only correctly established by scholarship in the 1950s [Laslett, 1963].) It also paved the way for the establishment of a much more limited, constitutional monarchy that shared power with parliament. These are hallmarks in the development of liberal democracy, and Locke was the great theorist of them.

Locke's sovereign, which he did not identify with the monarch or the aristocracy, but with the majority of the people (i.e., those males who owned property and had a right to vote), does not need to be as unlimited or powerful as Hobbes's because for him the natural condition is not as dire. Locke's state of nature has two stages. The first stage is a scene of personal freedom and self-sovereignty but checked by natural reason that led most men to be peaceable and cooperative most of the time. Locke's state of nature is not a place where reason is self-defeating, but it does lack impartial referees to enforce common rules for living. The rules, themselves, are moral, unwritten, and rather vague. But because there is abundance in physical nature, a reasonable basis for limited trust and secure future planning, and natural fairness, the first stage of the state of nature is able to do without absolute sovereignty or, indeed, without government of any kind. In the second stage of the state of nature, conflict breaks out due to developing inequality and artificial scarcity. Locke attributes this to the invention of money.

Before money, in a natural barter economy, individuals appropriate only as much as they could use without spoilage. There is no way to stockpile and preserve natural consumable goods, and because anyone could easily return to the natural stockpile at any time, there is no self-interested reason to hoard or to try to seize another's resources. When goods could be transformed into a durable form of money, unlimited accumulation became reasonable and, in fact, highly desirable. This leads to conflict and to the establishment of government in order to provide impartial arbitrators to resolve disputes, to set rules for the protection of private property and the promotion of commerce, and to manage production and distribution in the political economy. Locke paid much more attention to the exploitation and appropriation of physical nature or environmental resources than did Hobbes and Rousseau.

Jean-Jacques Rousseau (1712–1778)

In many ways, Rousseau's thinking about the state of nature and the social contract was closer to Hobbes's than to Locke's, but as a latecomer to the traditional discourse of social contract theory he could critically position himself in relation to each of his predecessors. Rousseau believed that Hobbes had improperly projected conflict that is the product of social existence onto natural existence.

Likewise, he thought Locke projected reason and a form of morality (external natural laws and the inner capacity to understand and obey them, conscience) mistakenly onto the state of nature, when what he is really describing is a state of society of a certain kind. Rousseau was determined to reach back to bare nature, but what he found there was essentially human absence. Both conflict and orderly moral and social living were part of a narrative of movement from the natural state to the social state—each possibilities of humanness, neither essential nor inherent.

In his main work of political philosophy, an incomplete and rather cryptic book entitled *On the Social Contract* (*Du contrat social*), he presents his conception of the motivational and moral basis of sovereign authority in a human political culture. Like Hobbes, he probes deeply into the psychological and ontological sources of sovereign power as the only alternative to insecurity, conflict, mean living, and death. Locke anticipates the later work of theorists in the liberal tradition in that his main concern was liberty and fairness and impartial justice. Like Hobbes, Rousseau played for more basic stakes, life itself and the natural and social conditions of life's flourishing.

Hobbes saw sovereignty embedded in political institutions—monarchy, aristocracy, or democracy—and the establishment of sovereign authority grew out of a reciprocal agreement, every man with every man, to have their private wills represented by and become subordinate to the will of the sovereign representative. Rousseau saw sovereignty as what he called the "general will." This is not a person or an office; it is a moral culture and a spirit of community and solidarity. It is a capacity for moral imagination and agency (hence, "will") informed by a widespread sense of common need, vulnerability, and equal concern and respect. The general will stands behind all other forms of legitimate rule and power in a society. It is socially and politically embodied in a participatory republic, a set of interlocking governance institutions that rest on the periodic re-creation of the general will by a popular assembly of all citizens. And the general will is culturally embedded in a special form of moral will and moral imagination, one informed by the independent judgment of each citizen and by a strong awareness of mutual need and vulnerability, in which, to borrow a phrase from Marx, whose core idea was already present in Rousseau, the free development of each depends on the free development of all. It is a rare, difficult, and precarious achievement in human history, but it is the highest expression of our communal humanity, and it arises out of the development of humanity out of nature and through culture.

Unlike Hobbes in *Leviathan* and Locke in the *Two Treatises of Government,* Rousseau does not present all the elements of his version of social contract theory in a single work. In *On the Social Contract,* he tries to give the contractarian dialectic of nature and culture a kind of rigorous, logical form. There he delights in showing the inconsistencies and false inferences of other modes of theory and political reasoning. His interesting and original account of the state of nature is cast as a conjecture about the phylogenetic development of humanness and the origins of social inequality, and it is set out most fully in his *Discourse on the Origins and Foundations of Inequality among Men.* Finally, essential to Rousseau's understanding of nature and culture is *Émile,* a hybrid work, part novel and part educational manual, that is the counterpart of the *Discourse on Inequality* only cast on the ontogenetic level, in the *bildung* of Émile from infancy to adulthood, from natural animal to natural man.

In these and other works, Rousseau showed not only the logical acumen on display in *On the Social Contract,* but a remarkable critical eye as a social and cultural observer of the society of the last years of the French ancien régime.[1] The central concept of his cultural and social criticism was *amour propre,* meaning vanity, self-regard, the tendency to get one's sense of self from the eyes and approval of others, insincerity, inauthenticity, narcissism. As amour propre came to dominate the identity and motivation of modern man, it became the driving force behind injustice, conflict, and the eclipse of true moral individuality and citizenship behind the security providing power of Hobbesian sovereignty and subjection.

A Logic of Nature and Culture

Social contract theory explicitly rests on a contrast between a cultural and a natural form of life or condition of existence. The natural condition, which is commonly called the state of nature, is used both as a vehicle for presenting the theory's conception of what is rooted in (human) nature and as a heuristic construct that clarifies the essential features of the cultural condition, both the normative, ideal cultural conditions and deformed, unjust ones.

In social contract theories, the natural state of being is mainly interesting for what it lacks and as a way of instructing us about the human consequences of that lack. What it lacks, of course, are precisely those features that at least partially define the cultural state of being and the consequences of that lack are what the transition from the natural to the cultural condition is supposed to remedy.[2]

To perform this theoretical function, it is not necessary for nature to be conceived in isolation from the human. John Stuart Mill once defined nature as everything that remains if human being and doing were taken away (1985). For the seventeenth- and eighteenth-century contractarians, the state of nature has many social and cultural elements built into it. Rousseau complained about this but then reproduced a nuanced version of the same thing into his own theorizing. For all social contract theorists, including Rousseau, those elements that are said to be absent in nature are carefully selected to reinforce and illustrate the theorist's view of what is most important about cultural order. The state of nature is often a construct used as a critical mirror held up against a particular culture or political system.

Generally speaking, the defining features of "the cultural" are the systematic and institutionalized organization of power and authority; the system of orderly coordination and cooperation among large numbers of individuals; and the sense of membership and common interest. In short, the absence in nature is an absence of form—institutional form and psychological or motivational form. It is an absence of that which is necessary to channel, coordinate, and contain the remarkably broad agency of the human animal. *Homo sapiens* is a creature propelled by drives and reasons, but not much by instinct, a creature with a remarkably wide behavioral repertoire and an extraordinarily flexible adaptive capacity. Nature is semantics without syntax, speech without grammar, symphony without score.

Social contract theory is a story about the process of *civil*-ization and human self-realization. The move from the natural to the cultural is a move forward, from a condition of moral and social isolation (Rousseau turned this into true solitude, Hobbes and Locke did not) to sociality and interdependence; the human is the domain of mutual need and assistance. It is logically possible, I suppose, to reverse the direction of this evaluative arrow.[3] The state of nature's lack of cultural things may be taken as a sign of plenitude rather than deprivation; the transition from the natural to the cultural may be seen as a fall rather than as an advance.

Although this interpretation of the transition from nature to culture as a fall is logically possible, it is out of keeping with the genre of social contract theorizing. The story told in the contractarian narrative does not lend itself to either primitivism or anarchism. Bare nature, which has not yet reached culture or full humanness, is depicted as both primitive and anarchistic, politically headless because it is not yet politically and culturally minded. The currents of thought in the social contract apparatus run against this condition; primitivism and anarchism are signs of cultural absence, not cultural plenitude and humanizing meaning. To render them culturally fulfilling requires a different kind of narrative, a narrative of mythic origins or an evolutionary story of cooperation and altruism, such as is found in Kropotkin.

However, Rousseau does do something novel in that he offers two very different accounts of the founding social contract—the contractarian moment, as it were. In the *Discourse on Inequality* he construes a phony social contract in which the wealthy few dupe the simple many. This is a fall not from what he counts as man's natural condition but from what he calls the "Golden Age," an already rich and complex cultural order that contains the elements of transparency, justice, love, community, and empathy he is looking for in the authentic social contract.[4] The authentic contract, outlined abstractly in *On the Social Contract* and summarized in *Émile,* consolidates and protects the human virtues of the Golden Age, much as the phony contract poisons and eventually transmutes them into pride, vanity, greed, the will to power, duplicity, insincerely, and loss of true self.

However the theorist may flesh out and manipulate nature and culture, a common element in social contract theory is its critical power. This critical power has three aspects. First, as has been noted, social contract theory motivates the human story through a critique of the absence of form in its conceptualization of nature. The raw material of humanness is there, but the shape it can take has yet to be determined. Second, it presents an ideal conception of human affirmation in a just cultural order that is founded by the social contract. Finally, it mounts a critique of presently existing social and political order by way of contrast—the existing order does not remedy the deficiencies of nature, or it distorts nature's possibilities. The existing order fails to embody the ideals and purposes animating the aboriginal founding, and thus it fundamentally lacks legitimacy and authority. It rests on a deception and a kind of misdirection of the human story (*bildung*). When a social contract theory lays out what it takes to be the appropriate general form of cultural being, it thereby establishes an evaluative standard, a regulative ideal, against which any particular existing cultural arrangements can be judged.

Here contractarian theory takes an interesting departure from Aristotelianism, stoicism, and earlier forms of natural law theory, out of which contractarianism directly emanated. These theories took nature itself to be the source of ethical and political regulative ideals; culture then was to be molded in nature's image. Contractarianism uses the interplay between nature and culture to capture a radically different phenomenon: not the molding of culture by nature, but the human creation of value through a kind of dialectic of nature and culture. In that dialectic nature is reconstituted through culture, and culture recovers nature in order to sustain itself. I shall say more about this dialectic of nature and culture below.

The Inner and the Outer

Thus far I have been emphasizing how the outer order of humanity—social, cultural, and political order—can be evaluated in the mirror of nature. Social contract theory can also develop an analogous critical perspective on the inner order of humanity—psychological, motivational, aesthetic, and intellectual order. Again, in regard to inner form, the state of nature is more theoretically illuminating by dint of what it lacks than what it contains, and its use as a negative heuristic device, so to speak, can be applied to the theory's underlying conception of well-realized humanity or the human good. When it is so applied, social contract theory provides a powerful conceptual framework for distinguishing between what is exclusively natural in humans (man-in-the-state-of-nature, or the "mere condition of nature," as Hobbes put it) and humanized nature or "second nature," which is the natural cultivated. I say cultivated, not subdued, replaced, or turned into sheer artifice, because I am struck by the deliberateness of the contractarian thinkers in seeing the cultural state of humanness as *accommodating and building on* natural tendencies and potentialities, which nature alone is unable to bring to fruition in human beings, not as *creating and controlling* those tendencies and potentialities out of whole cloth.

Nonetheless, within this impulse to build on rather than to replace nature in order to achieve humanity (that is to say, in order to achieve a cultural ecology in which humanity can flourish), two significantly different emphases are possible. This difference, in my estimation, is one of the most important things separating Hobbes and Rousseau. For Hobbes, to move from the state of nature into cultural order is to change the behavioral manifestations of the natural in mankind by changing the environment in which that nature expresses itself. For Rousseau, the transition from nature to culture is a qualitative transformation of the natural.

Let me try to formulate this in a slightly different way. For Hobbes, the inner order of humanity was complete and given already in nature—only the outer, cultural order of properly realized humanity was naturally absent. Humans lurking in ambush in the state of nature (or state of war) are not fundamentally different creatures from what they are when they walk securely and confidently in the streets of Leviathan state.

For Rousseau, by contrast, humanity is in ontological motion. This applies to human beings both as they (potentially) exist in the state of nature and as they (actually) exist in civil society. The human lies at the intersection of the natural and the cultural, and it is dynamic and perfectible. Right cultural order is to be evaluated both by the plenitude it offers in the face of nature's absences and by the extent to which it serves as a developmental medium for the evolution of inner nature. It is not altogether easy to say how this transformation should be characterized. Rousseau often resorts to paradoxical formulations, for example in *Émile* where he is at pains to show that it takes a great deal of artifice to make man natural. There is something inherent in the right kind of interaction between nature and culture that transcends the qualities in either of the interacting components. Culture can build on and bring out the good in nature; it can create virtue and the moral will, just as it can also bring out the worst in humanity, a deformed and improperly realized humanness. But nature also brings out the good in culture. Neither concept points to a state of being sufficient and perfect unto itself. Only in their interaction do we find the good state of human being.

This gives Rousseau's thought tremendous hermeneutical interest, and many philosophical difficulties. Again, I would turn our attention to the tension between what a theorist wants to say and the conceptual vocabulary available to him or her for saying it. Rousseau was a developmental contractarian, and that is just short of an oxymoron. He took a theoretical apparatus that deploys fundamental categories like nature and culture in such a way that the good is driven by the evil at its back, and he tried to use it to convey a vision of the good beckoned by the best that stands on a horizon before it.

Why is it preferable to say that culture perfects nature rather than that it merely uses nature or provides a new context for nature? Those contractarians, like Hobbes, who resist the notion that man becomes more fully human in becoming cultural encounter difficulties of their own. For if human self-realization is not at stake in the transition from the state of nature to cultural society, if this transition remedies no ontological lack in humanity (although it does remedy a lack in human transactions), then the stakes simply cannot be as high, nor the cultural telos as compelling, as they are for a contractarian such as Rousseau. And, short of the realization of a higher form of human excellence, what other ends can impel mankind out of the state of nature and justify the cultural order put in its place? Contractarians must struggle to find a good answer to this question.

The Dialectic of Nature and Culture

Hobbes and Rousseau were at pains to understand fundamental cultural issues—particularly the nature and limits of liberty and authority within a just cultural order—in the light of an underlying philosophical conception of human nature. Yet, at least for Rousseau, human nature was not an essence; it was not a set of timeless and universal properties that establish the parameters of cultural and moral possibility.

The becoming that takes us from nature to culture is a transformation that constitutes humanity. It can be a transformation in which, through culture, human being is either elevated above nature or degraded beneath it. In a move anticipated, but not pushed as far, by Hobbes, Rousseau recasts the traditional idea of a human nature or essence that is timeless and universal into human nature as the developmental emergence of humanity out of the dialectical interplay of the natural and the cultural. Properly realized or well-formed humanity (marked by motivations of civic virtue and the moral will) grows out of the cultural and political structures he sketched in *On the Social Contract.* Improperly realized or deformed humanity (marked by amour propre, insecure and duplicitous identity and strategically self-regarding and manipulative behavior) grew out of the social and technological features of modernity, although its roots lie as far back as the invention of private property, the environmental exploitations associated with agriculture and mining, and even with the origins of language itself, and hence the origins of self-consciousness and imagination.

Hobbes and Rousseau opened a new chapter in the history of cultural thought, and it is a chapter cultural theorists are still writing, although many intellectual winds have shifted away from this style of philosophical humanism. Hobbes and Rousseau gave discourse about nature, not simply a place, but the fundamental place in their cultural theories. Their work represents a culmination of the natural law tradition and points beyond it to the wholly secular conception of man and society that has been the hallmark of cultural and social theory since the French Revolution, notably in the modern development of the social sciences. Hobbes and Rousseau developed conceptions of the natural foundations of cultural order that were independent of any transcendent metaphysics, cosmology, or theology. They maintained that cultural order is the artificial, rational construction of human will. But they went even further and argued that in constructing cultural order, human beings have no transcendent pattern to follow.

Without the benefit of transcendent reason or revelation, man becomes not simply the constructor of cultural order but, in a much more radical sense, its creator—not the architect of order but its author. And the blueprints, as well as the raw materials, for this creation have to come from within its creators, from what humanity inherits from nature.

Moreover, if man is the creator of cultural order in an ontological sense, the practical task facing particular men and women who must create and sustain— produce and reproduce—a particular cultural order requires that they too must look inward and outward rather than upward for guidance. The kind of radical cultural creativity entailed by contractarian theories like those of Hobbes and Rousseau requires a radical and exacting kind of self-knowledge by cultural agents.

Hobbes, whose theory is logically indifferent as to the institutional form the sovereign may take, preferred the form with (he thought) the greatest centripetal force, namely, monarchy. Conceived as a representative person, the Hobbesian sovereign needs only to be able to read himself, but in a particular and demanding way: to read in himself mankind and to read mankind in himself. *Leviathan* was written to teach him (but who?) to do precisely this. In order to succeed, *Leviathan* had to find only one reader, but how much more difficult is that task than achieving sales in the millions?

To successfully ground his more participatory and democratic conception of the ideal cultural order, Rousseau had somehow to extend the diffusion of this culturally creative self-knowledge more widely than did Hobbes. The viability of the Rousseauian cultural order demands a more positive, active, and energetic mode of citizenship by a greater number of individual members of the cultural community than the Hobbesian cultural order demands for its viability. These differences are real and important, but they should not be permitted to obscure an equally fundamental element that binds Hobbes and Rousseau together in a common theoretical enterprise.

This common element is what I referred to earlier as the dialectic of nature and culture. In order to develop this notion more fully, consider the following four propositions:

First, the natural condition of mankind is a radically individualistic condition of absolute liberty, equality, and self-sovereignty. (For Hobbes this leads to a war of all against all that negates most of the advantages of our humanness; for Rousseau this leads to a serene and scattered peace among creatures who carry within themselves the co-evolutionary possibilities of mutual war or communal justice.) Cultural order is conventional or artificial; there is no transcendent principle of moral duty that impels or obliges human beings to leave their natural, precultural condition and enter into a cultural mode of existence. To be sure, Hobbes adumbrates what he calls the "laws of nature," but they are not binding in the state of nature and have moral force only after the institution of sovereign authority, not before. Unless, Hobbes adds, surely tongue in cheek, one views God as the sovereign and the laws of nature as his civil edicts. Likewise for Rousseau, there is no morality, and no need for morality, in the state of nature. He gives a pre-Darwinian, but nonetheless naturalistic and evolutionary, account of how the movement from nature to culture can be explained. For this we need a narrative form of explanation appropriate to natural and human history, not the nomothetic-deductive type of explanation used in the nonhistorical natural sciences. In my opinion, Rousseau's account is a richer and more suggestive speculative reconstruction than contemporary sociobiologists or evolutionary psychologists have managed to concoct (Fodor and Piattelli-Palmarini 2010).

Second, human nature—considered as a complex of rational capacities, passionate drives, and inherent potentialities—provides the starting point for the emergence of humanity as both inner psychic order and outer cultural order constitute it. But the possibilities of our nature will always exceed the actualities of our realized humanness. Thus, social contract theory, at least as Hobbes and Rousseau fashion it, has an element of tragedy. Whatever cultural condition of life is built on it, human beings will be marked by estrangement from nature. Even properly realized humanity in a virtuous and just culture will be a kind of "denaturing." Natural humanity and civic humanity (man and citizen) do not completely coincide or overlap.

For Hobbes, that estrangement is endemic and ontological—being is matter in motion; living being is metabolic in the sense that it has a basic impulse, the "endeavor" toward self-preservation; and the experience of being human is "a restless desire of power after power that ceases only in death," as Hobbes put it in the important eleventh chapter of *Leviathan* (1946, p. 64). For Rousseau, the sources of this estrangement are both ontogenetic and phylogenetic. At the individual level, it resides in the betrayals of infancy and childhood, malicious (as a boy, Rousseau was locked outside the gate of Geneva by a malign gatekeeper who deliberately, Rousseau thought, closed them early) or inadvertent (Rousseau's mother died in childbirth and thus he remarks, "my birth was the first of my misfortunes" [1954, p. 19]). At the species level, it resides in the fatal rise of self-consciousness and imagination that is inseparable from the acquisition of language, and with it distinctions between self and other, mine and yours.

Third, although necessarily alienating to some degree, a just cultural order— culture as a "corrected fullness," to borrow Sheldon Wolin's (2004, p. 19) apt phrase, mitigating nature's absences—does constitute the most fully human mode of existence. But to be viable and sustainable, any cultural order must be compatible with the psychological possibilities determined by human nature. Of any contractarian theory ask: Does the political psychology on which the theory is premised plausibly enable the reproduction over time of the civic motivation that a just cultural order needs to sustain itself and its politics? Hobbesian natural men become citizens by the push of fear and advantage. But surely citizens are needed most precisely when it is vital to overcome fear and advantage, when the push of self-interest must give way to the pull of moral ideals. Rousseauian natural men become corrupt cultural men by duplicity and by the triumph of amour propre over *pitié* (compassion, care, spontaneous aversion to suffering). Fully modern and corrupt cultural men cannot become citizens. But those in the back-waters or byways of modernity (like the Genevans or the Corsicans), or those specially tutored (like Émile), may become citizens (or at least become fit for citizenship should they find a just republic to join) by returning to the sources of morality anterior to reason in nature (*amour-de-soi* and *pitié*, but not amour propre) and reconstructing them in artificial form, or in the form of their "second nature" as moral will and civic virtue. Notice that, for both Hobbes and Rousseau, nature is not constituted by reason; reason is a component of culture. For Hobbes, reason is merely the capacity to relate desired ends to efficient means; rational thoughts, as he put it, "are to the desires, as scouts, and spies, to range abroad, and find the way to the things desired" (1946, part 1, chap. 8, p. 46). For Rousseau, nature is constituted by love, and the basic story of the development of humanity through culture, man's self-becoming, is the story of the appropriate or inappropriate cultural apprehension of natural love in cultural and political form.

Fourth, the contingent conditions of human temporal and earthly existence are made up of material relationships with the objects of the physical and biological environment, relationships limited by biological and thermodynamic parameters and mediated by technology, social organization, and grammars of symbolic or semiotic meaning. These contingent conditions of human natural existence elect and make manifest some, but never all, of the immanent possibilities of nature and humanity. These material and social relationships thus construct a realized human nature—that is, a specific repertoire of rationality, emotion, motivation, will, meaningful agency, and behavior—and a cultural order embodied in place and embedded in time.

This structure of ideas indicates how complex matters become when theorists recognize (as Rousseau did more adequately than Hobbes) that the culturally pertinent psychological traits of human beings are themselves the products of both nature and culture and must be understood in light of both. The paradox noted above arises because a naturalistic interpretation of these traits presupposes a cultural interpretation of them and vice versa. For Hobbes, these psychological traits are essential and timeless, but they manifest themselves only contingently and culturally according to a logic of strategic patterns of social interaction. For Rousseau, the inner order of humanity is potentially given in nature but has two possible destinies: a virtuous communal and moral one or a corrupt one of competitive and possessive individualism.

In sum, the cultural theories of Hobbes and Rousseau involve an exceedingly complex dialectic of nature and culture, played out simultaneously in the inner world of reason, passion, motivation, and will and in the outer world of cultural action, authority, liberty, and obedience. In varying degrees, both Hobbes and Rousseau recognized that their efforts to push the logic of social contract theory to its limits had led their thought to become caught up in conundrums from which it could not escape.

One escape, perhaps the only one possible, came by way of Kant, who fell more or less back on a transcendental dualism, not the substantive ontological dualism of Descartes (Todes, 2001), and abandoned the quest for a philosophy in which nature and culture could mirror, challenge, compliment, and supplement one another. The nineteenth century and early twentieth century buried contractarian theory of the pre-Kantian variety and was torn between idealism and a number of rather less subtle naturalisms.[5] With the late-twentieth-century revival of contractarian theory, by the time we come to Rawls or Gauthier, the themes with which I have been concerned are not central to what is most interesting about these theories.

To find the real heirs of the type of theoretical project I have tried to explore briefly and abstractly in the work of Hobbes and Rousseau, one must turn to Marx and to Freud, each of whom explored the interplay of nature and culture using a theoretical discourse and conceptual apparatus quite different from Hobbes and Rousseau, yet the echoes of Hobbes in Freud, and of Rousseau in Marx, are palpable. At this time, both of these strong readers of nature and culture are in eclipse, which shocks me when I think back to how fundamental and central they were to my own education and intellectual formation. With them, this entire paradigm of discourse has fallen silent, more or less, its place taken by genomics and neuroscience, by evolutionary psychology and "evo-devo" (evolutionary developmental biology). That some of these modes of discourse and theory will prove rich in a certain way, I have no doubt (see Wheeler, 2006; Connolly, 2002). But I do confess that I will be grateful when this current period of philosophical and intellectual amnesia comes to an end. Then perhaps we can return in a rigorous and straightforward way to a philosophical humanism that engages the categories of nature, culture, and humanity to their full effect and in their complex interdependent meanings.

NOTES

1. It should be noted that Rousseau was a significant naturalist, in addition to being a social philosopher, novelist, playwright, composer, and autobiographer. He wrote widely on botany and on various landscapes, stressing the moral and spiritual effects of living within environments of undisturbed natural beauty.

2. The defining features of "the natural" in social contract theory are not those that have been emphasized in connection with "the primitive" or "the savage" in nineteenth-century social anthropology—preliterate communication, nonabstract and nonscientific or animistic modes of thought, technologically simple hunting and gathering economies with small band organization and little impact on the ecosystems they inhabit beyond the carrying capacity of those systems. See Lévy-Bruhl (1966). See also Diamond (1974), Clarke and Hindley (1975), and Kunstler (2006). For critical perspectives on this body of thought, see Lévi-Strauss (1966), Sahlins, (1977), and Meek (1976).

3. For versions of contract theory that move in the direction of anarchism, see Wolff (1970) and Nozick (1974). Illuminating discussions of the nature and logic of

contract theory can be found in Nozick and in the work of David Gauthier (1969; 1977; 1986).

4. The notion of the Golden Age was well established in Ovid and other classical sources and was a familiar rhetorical convention in Rousseau's time. Among many examples that could be cited, see the remarkable depiction of the Golden Age in *Don Quixote,* part 1, chapter 11 (Cervantes Saavedra, 2003, pp. 76–78).

5. The history of philosophical anthropology after Kant tends to be centered in Germany and involves a split between two influential schools of Neo-Kantianism, the so-called South-western School and the Marburg School, exemplified by two great philosophers in this field, Wilhelm Dilthey and Ernst Cassirer, respectively. Cf. Skidelsky (2008), Barash (2008), and Gordon (2010).

REFERENCES

Barash, J. A., ed. 2008. *The Symbolic Construction of Reality: The Legacy of Ernst Cassirer.* Chicago: University of Chicago Press.
Cervantes Saavedra, M. 2003. *Don Quixote.* Trans. E. Grossman. New York: Harper Collins.
Clarke, R., and G. Hindley. 1975. *The Challenge of the Primitives.* New York: McGraw-Hill.
Connolly, W. E. 2002. *Neuropolitics: Thinking, Culture, Speed.* Minneapolis: University of Minnesota Press.
Diamond, M. 1974. *In Search of the Primitive.* New Brunswick, N.J.: Transaction.
Fodor, J., and M. Piattelli-Palmarini. 2010. *What Darwin Got Wrong.* New York: Farrar, Strauss and Giroux.
Gauthier, D. 1969. *The Logic of Leviathan.* Oxford: Oxford University Press.
———. 1977. "The Social Contract as Ideology." *Philosophy and Public Affairs* 6 (Winter): 130–64.
———. 1986. *Morals by Agreement.* New York: Oxford University Press.
Gordon, P. E. 2010. *Continental Divide: Heidegger, Cassirer, Davos.* Cambridge, Mass.: Harvard University Press.
Hobbes, T. 1946. *Leviathan.* Ed. M. Oakeshott. Oxford: Basil Blackwell.
Hirschman, A. O. 1991. *The Rhetoric of Reaction.* Cambridge, Mass.: Harvard University Press.
Kunstler, J. H. 2006. *The Long Emergency: Surviving the End of Oil, Climate Change, and Other Converging Catastrophes of the Twenty-First Century.* New York: Grove.
Laslett, P. 1963. Introduction to *John Locke Two Treatises of Government,* rev. ed. Cambridge: Cambridge University Press, pp. 15–168.
Lévi-Strauss, C. 1966. *The Savage Mind.* Chicago: University of Chicago Press.
Lévy-Bruhl, L. 1966. *Primitive Mentality.* Boston: Beacon.
Meek, R. L. 1976. *Social Science and the Ignoble Savage.* New York: Cambridge University Press.
Mill, J. S. 1985. "Nature." In *The Collected Works of John Stuart Mill,* vol. 10, *Essays on Ethics, Religion, and Society,* ed. John M. Robson, pp. 373–402. Toronto: University of Toronto Press, London: Routledge & Kegan Paul.

Nozick, R. 1974. *Anarchy, State, and Utopia.* New York: Basic Books.

Pocock, J. G. A. 1973. *Politics, Language, and Time.* New York: Atheneum.

Rousseau, J. J. 1954. *Confessions.* Trans. J. M. Cohen. Harmondsworth, U.K.: Penguin.

———. 1978. *On the Social Contract, with Geneva Manuscript and Political Economy.* Ed. R. D. Masters. Trans. J. R. Masters. New York: St. Martin's.

Sahlins, M. 1977. *Culture and Practical Reason.* Chicago: University of Chicago Press.

Skidelsky, E. 2008. *Ernst Cassirer: The Last Philosopher of Culture.* Princeton: Princeton University Press.

Todes, S. 2001. *Body and World.* Cambridge, Mass.: MIT Press.

Wheeler, W. 2006. *The Whole Creature: Complexity, Biosemiotics, and the Evolution of Culture.* London: Lawrence & Wishart.

Wolff, R. P. 1970. *In Defense of Anarchism.* New York: Harper & Row.

Wolin, S. S. 2004. *Politics and Vision: Innovation and Continuity in Western Political Thought.* Expanded ed. Princeton: Princeton University Press.

CHAPTER FOUR

Human Nature without Theory

Gregory E. Kaebnick, Ph.D.

The feeling is by no means universal, but a decent-sized swath of the public thinks that what people might someday be able to do to modify human bodies using biotechnologies is at odds with some of their attitudes about the moral significance of human nature. Exactly how to describe these attitudes and exactly what "at odds" means lead into murky waters, however. We do not know our way around when it comes to articulating our views about the moral significance of human nature. Thoughtful people sympathetic to these attitudes describe them only gropingly.

Critics have no trouble. Not infrequently, one can hear a moral concern about human nature outlined in the form of a quick and crude objection: "X is against nature, and therefore wrong."[1] In this rendering, the moral concern is simple, confident, forceful—and ridiculous. One of its more preposterous aspects is that "against nature" implies that we know what human nature is, when surely human nature is amorphous and slippery at best. The difficulty of pinning down human nature is one reason that attitudes about nature cannot be plausible unless they are limited and complicated.

In this chapter, I argue that we may not need to know much about human nature to have moral concerns about changing it by means of biotechnology. More precisely, I maintain that we do not need to have a full theory of human nature to have moral concerns about changing it. The concept "human nature" must refer to something in the real world if we are to attach moral significance to it, but we need not (so I argue) be able to say exactly what it means to be human.

The Concept of Human Nature

The moral concerns people have about human nature rest on different positions on the very concept of what human nature is—different views, that is to say, of what one knows when one has an understanding of human nature. Some of these positions would require a full theory of human nature, but others do not.

Essentialist versus Evolutionary Views of Species

According to one long and deep philosophical tradition, to have a concept of human nature is to grasp the essence of the ontological category that (in this account) human nature is. This would be more than a mere description; it would provide a metaphysical explanation of why things in that category belong to the category. It would set out the "what it is to be" of that thing, as Aristotle's language is sometimes translated.

Understanding the essence of human nature would amount to having a full theory of human nature. As typically understood, an "essence" is the concept that a particular thing embodies. The essence of a triangle, for example, is the definition of triangles that all particular triangles embody. The essence of gold is the molecular structure that characterizes gold. An essence explains the traits that a thing has. It is not reducible to those traits, however; it is unchanging and timeless. An essence has an existence of its own, and indeed it is, in a sense, more real than the items that partake of it. Further, essences are often held to relate things of different kinds to each other. An essence is unique; all the members of a given kind share an essence, and members of other kinds lack it. According to an ancient lineage of scholars whose work draws on Aristotle, the universe reflects God's benevolent organization—a "great chain of being," so to speak, of essences is often invoked to suggest that a kind is what it is by rational necessity and that the overall universe is also rationally ordered and necessary. We understand the order and necessity of the universe by grasping the essences that things in the universe embody.

This is a lot to take on. Fortunately, essentialism is not the only way of understanding the concept of "human nature." Essentialism models itself after mathematics and physics, but biology is now understood along evolutionary and stridently nonessentialist lines. The evolutionary view makes no claim for the rational necessity of human nature, or for its immutability and timelessness, or that an account of human nature will show that human nature is rationally re-lated to the rest of the universe. There need also be no requirement that what makes humans human is some trait that the members of other species entirely lack. Typically, looking at traits allows one to recognize species, but the traits that allow us to recognize humans as humans might all be found in some measure in other animals. And ultimately, in an evolutionary account, what really distin-guishes species is not any claim about what traits characterize the members of the species, but the causal story that can be told about how the species appeared on the scene and how, through reproduction, it persists. In an evolutionary account, whether a given population of animals really counts as a "species" can be allowed to remain somewhat problematic and contestable.

If the evolutionary view of species makes sense, then the term "human nature" does not demarcate the set—it does not show what counts as a human being and what does not. Instead, it functions descriptively; it tells us what the members of the set happen to be like. Of course, because evolutionary stories are also stories about how species came to be *what* they are, we expect to be able to talk knowl-edgeably both about traits that distinguish species from each other and about traits that species share—to describe, for example, how dogs and cats are similar and how they differ. In the evolutionary view, this is to talk about species' natures.

Talk about what dogs, cats, and other kinds of animals are like is unproblem-atic. And because humans are themselves animals—and *only* animals, in a Dar-winian frame—then we should expect to be able to talk about human nature. Moreover, we should expect to make some headway in understanding human nature by studying our taxonomic neighbors, as Mary Midgley argues in *Beast and Man* (1979). What distinguishes human beings from other animals is typi-cally held to be their possession of various capacities related to cognition, such as language, rationality, tool-making, morality, and culture, but there is no need to establish that any of these capacities are possessed *only* by humans; indeed, the evidence is mounting that they are capacities or extensions of capacities that ani-mals also possess in differing forms and degrees. At the same time, as Midgley also emphasizes, we need not restrict ourselves to biology to learn about human nature. We will have to study humans sociologically and anthropologically, as Paul Ehrlich (2000) does in arguing that there is no unitary account of human nature, and in favor of thinking that, given the significance of culture in human ways of living, there are multiple human natures.

Thinking this way leads to lists, while also ensuring that any one list will be less than completely satisfying. Larry Arnhart offers a list of twenty natural desires "that are so deeply rooted in human nature that they will manifest themselves in some manner in every human society" (1998, p. 29). Martha Nussbaum offers ten "central capabilities" that represent "a type of *overlapping consensus* on the part of people with otherwise very different views of human life" (2000, p. 76). Such lists often seem to be on to something; at the same time, they sometimes seem pat and open to quibbling. Arnhart includes sexuality on his list; Nussbaum subsumes it under "bodily integrity." Nussbaum includes "affiliation," Arnhart "relationships" but also the more explicitly community-minded "sociality." Nussbaum includes "life" and "bodily health" but not "embodiment" per se, as Leon Kass certainly would. In short, questions arise that can look like matters of judgment: Why is *this* left off? Is *that* really a general feature of human nature? Why not break that one into two items? Arnhart notes that the items on the list need not be true of every individual; it is enough that they are "tendencies or proclivities" that are manifest on the population level (1998, p. 30). And both Arnhart and Nussbaum observe that the items may be instantiated very differently in different societies. We must see all such lists as open to challenge and revision. Nussbaum emphasizes this point: "the list remains open-ended and humble; it can always be contested and remade" (2000, p. 77).

Another broader point must be made here: what the term "nature" means in general also depends on our interests and on the conceptual frame within which we are operating. John Stuart Mill famously sought to dismiss the thought that "nature" can have intrinsic moral value by showing that it refers to many different things, many of them undesirable, and that the two most common ways of understanding "nature" can give no moral direction. Under one common understanding, "nature" refers to everything that adheres to the laws of nature; under the other, it refers only to that which excludes human interference or involvement. Understood in the first way, all human action is natural; understood the second way, all human action is unnatural. Either way, the concept cannot help us mark off *some* human actions as according with nature and others as violating it (1961, pp. 368 ff.).

The response to Mill can only be to acknowledge the complexity and work with it. When we are doing physics, everything that is, is natural. When we are shopping for food, deciding where to spend a vacation, or arguing about how national forests are maintained, we will see certain ways in which humans can manipulate the world around them as altering natural states of affairs. For the anthropologist and the cosmetic surgeon, perhaps everything that humans can do to themselves is natural. For the administrator of a sports league, certain things humans can do to themselves may not count as natural. Within these contexts, it will often be clear enough whether something counts as "natural," but we will also come up against situations in which we are not entirely sure how to carry on with the term, and we must adjudicate these hard cases as best we can, by appealing to standards developed within the context in which we are operating.

Norms versus Individual Differences

We would be committed to having a fairly complete account of human nature—though a more limited theory than essentialism implies—if understanding human nature means understanding species norms. We would be committed to having a well-supported account of what features make up human nature, but we would not necessarily need to set out the features that distinguish human beings from the things in other categories.

Often, when people have discussed the role that the concept of human nature plays in moral argument, they have thought that to speak of human nature is to speak of norms and that to value human nature is to value those norms. Some have invoked human nature to argue, for example, that people fall—and should fall—into two distinct sexes and that the members of those sexes have—and should conform to—typical forms of behavior, especially as concerns gender roles and sexuality. Others have opposed the concept of human nature because they see it as supporting just those uses.

If we subscribe to the essentialist understanding of species, then we have no option but to speak about species norms. In fact, any variation from the norms will raise awkward questions about whether the label "human" is still appropriate. But if we take the evolutionary tack, we have options. We can distinguish between different things that "natural" is taken to mean. "Natural" might mean "normal" or might mean, more simply and more fundamentally, "as we find it." If we are using the first sense, then it is *the kind* that we value, and deviations would be devalued. Individuals would acquire value by instantiating species norms. Under the second construal of "nature," however, we value individuals and diversity, and we value species norms, not in themselves, but simply because they, too, are important features of the world as we find it.

This gives us a lot to say in defense of human variation. There might be ways of defending homosexuality against those who think it intrinsically wrong (that is, wrong because unnatural) by appeal to species norms; homosexuality might turn out to be part of a normal distribution of human sexual nature (whether it does is both an empirical question and a question about where one draws lines through continuous statistical curves to demarcate "the norm"). Analogously, no one would say that people who are uncommonly good at athletic activity lie outside the range of normal human behavior (or that their behavior is inappropriate). But if we are interested in nature in the second way, we can also defend homosexuality more directly; we can say this is how some people find themselves in the world, and they should be who they are. I suspect many will share this intuition.[2]

We can say similar things about other aspects of human sexuality. Consider ambiguous genitalia and other intersex conditions. In the past, doctors have often taken immediate action to disambiguate these conditions, surgically altering children so that they would fall more plainly into the categories of male and female. That sort of action is driven at least in part by the first construal of nature. But if we are thinking along the lines of the second construal, we would likely say there is some value in leaving ambiguous genitalia just as they are, even though they are certainly atypical.

Valuing individuality will not make us blind to kinds and norms, and there will be situations in which we still need to talk about kinds. In arguing against enhancement in sports, for example, one would want to offer some assertions about the range of normal human functioning—the levels of erythropoietin one can typically expect to find in a person's blood, for example, or the sorts of cases in which a person could be said to have a testosterone deficiency (and the levels of testosterone that therapy should aim to achieve). But this is an indirect way of bringing norms into consideration. The starting point is nature in the second sense—that in which "nature" refers to what we find in the world, in all its individual diversity, rather than to species norms. The norms may be explicitly recognized as somewhat arbitrary cutoffs, not as *the correct understanding* of human nature. And it is what we find in the world that is the locus of value: the point of objections to enhancement is that if enhancement is allowed, then sport does not provide a way of celebrating natural—given—human gifts, as perfected and displayed through hard work and discipline (Murray, 2007).

People whose capacities lie outside the typical human may compel us to talk about norms for other reasons, even though speaking of norms is often problematic in this context because norms can be deployed as a way of stigmatizing and discriminating against people who fail to conform to them. A common theme among those who theorize about human disability is that we find a way of accepting and valuing "the anomalous, even the pathological, and [that] we must do so if we are to proceed with our varied lives in a satisfactory and satisfying manner."[3] This is not necessarily to say that human disability or difference is *desirable*, as if we ought to work to *achieve* it by creating disabilities (Asch, 2006, p. 248). It is to say only that there is *something* of value in *accepting* these differences if they have arisen "by nature."

Nussbaum argues that saying some people lack, by nature, certain typical human capacities—that they are "disabled"—can also give cover to stigmatization and discrimination. "The use of terms suggesting the inevitability and 'naturalness' of such impairments masks a refusal to spend enough money to change things on a large scale for people with impairments" (2000, p. 188). This may at times be true. But to show that a moral term is covertly used to justify bad behavior does not reveal a problem with the moral term itself; one can justify a kind of cruelty by emphasizing the importance of honesty. And, as Nussbaum herself notes, whether a variation in human capacity amounts to a disability is often a function of human decisions about the way society and its institutions are designed. To acknowledge this fact is to decouple questions about whether an impairment is acquired "by nature" and whether (for example) a building ought to be redesigned in order to make it more accessible to more people.

Formulating public policy that affects people with disabilities may nonetheless require reference to norms of human nature. Nussbaum's underlying concern in arguing against justifying disability by appeal to nature is that we not accept unjust ways of distributing resources. Justice, as she understands it, requires that we ensure that all human beings, to the extent possible, have the opportunity to develop the basic human capabilities, which demands a greater societal commitment to people born with certain kinds of differences—not a pat acceptance that nature stood in the way. But we can agree with this, while also recognizing some value in leaving natural human variation alone, even when it amounts to disability. If our moral values are ultimately all merely facets of a single general value, rather than a heterogeneous and incommensurable lot, then either human difference or justice must win out, without any loss of value. Deciding that justice requires us to strive to bring about normal human capacity, for example, could not leave a sense that there was any disvalue in eliminating human difference; the value of accepting human variation would have to completely disappear. If we think values are heterogeneous and incommensurable, however, we can admit a residual moral loss even while reliably preferring to bring people up to normal human capacity. And understanding the decision this way helps make sense of those cases in which many people do find value in leaving a human body alone. Many find interventions that merely normalize *appearance* and do not directly affect human capacity particularly troubling. Nussbaum herself holds that if severe disabilities could be permanently removed by means of genetic engineering, then they should be, but that conditions that, though disabling, leave open a real chance of achieving the crucial human capabilities, might not be (see 2006, p. 193).

In considering Mill's challenge about the meaning of "nature," I have argued that we could acknowledge the complexity and work with it. The tension between accepting human variation and promoting normal human capacities has to do with how moral *values* stack up against each other, but an uncertainty about the very concept of human nature underlies it. "Human nature" can refer both to how individual human capacities are acquired and to general claims about human capacities. Human bodies and faces tend to look so and so, and that is a fact of nature. But there is also a surprising degree of variation, and that, too, is a fact of nature. Plainly, there is no single, overarching definition of "nature" that applies to all of the ways in which the term is used and always shows clearly what the correct usage is. However, both in rejecting the essentialist understanding of "human nature" and in allocating only a limited role to assertions about human species norms, we shift the focus from general claims about what human beings are like to a recognition of diversity, complexity, and individual variation. To do so is to give up pretensions to a commanding knowledge of what human beings are really like.

The Value of Human Nature

The moral concerns people have about modifying human nature are also various. Like the different views about what a concept of human nature is, views about the connection between human nature and moral value can have diverse implications for what one knows about human nature.

Human Nature as Inviolable Ontological Category

It is here we find the argument that "X is against nature and therefore wrong." Language like "going against nature" or "violating nature" implies that a special sort of category mistake is being made—things are not being filed in their right places—and that making this category mistake has overriding moral ramifications. Other moral considerations are otiose. To make this kind of claim is to endorse an essentialist understanding of human nature, and therefore a full theory of human nature. But among those who have written sympathetically about the moral significance of human nature, no one in bioethics claims bluntly that something can be described as wrong because it is against nature.

Human Nature as the Basis for Morality

Another strong claim about the connection between human nature and moral values is that the concept of human nature represents the very foundation for morality. This claim, too, commits one to a strong understanding of human nature. Whether or not human nature is the basis for morality, many of our moral judgments would be unreliable if our understanding of human nature was erroneous or incomplete. If we recommend punishment because we believe that it helps people rehabilitate themselves, but that belief is mistaken, then our judgments about punishment are unreliable. Our values lead to specific moral positions only in light of premises concerning relevant facts. But if human nature is the basis for morality, then our moral judgments may be wrong not only on factual premises but on values premises as well. Thus, to the extent we think we know what our values are, we must have a command of human nature.

We would also need a full theory of human nature if we wanted to draw a general moral line between enhancement and therapy—to assert that enhancement is always wrong. To establish that strong conclusion, we would need an account of what enhancement and therapy are. Perhaps we would try to show, for example, that enhancement refers to interventions that move individuals beyond human nature, and therapy to interventions that preserve or return individuals to human nature. To show that those definitions make sense, and then to be able to put them to use and place different interventions in the appropriate categories, we would need an account of human nature. For example, we might try to argue that human nature refers to species-typical functioning.

Leon Kass is often thought to provide a clear example of this way of thinking about the moral relevance of human nature and about human enhancement. Kass himself explicitly denies this view (2004, p. 296). Moreover, his method is not what one would expect if this were his view. The natural method for basing moral guidance directly on human nature would be first to set out an account of human nature and then to apply it as needed, but Kass's method is typically to start by considering questions of meaning. In a chapter about the creation of human embryos in the laboratory, the philosophical discussion begins with a section subtitled "The Meaning of the Question," and Kass explains that his "orientation" is "that before deciding what to do, one should try to understand the implications of doing or not doing" (p. 85). Kass then connects these, not to an account of human nature, which would offer various claims about what humans *are,* but to the "idea of humanness," which is a question of how we think about ourselves—a topic for poetry as much as for science.

This method seems to commit Kass only to a limited theory of human nature. He is making claims about what is species-typical for humans, but the claims do not amount to a complete account of what is human and what falls outside the category. Moreover, many of the claims he offers are about such basic features of human life—sexual procreation, growing old, and passing away—that they encompass not only all humans but all animals. Kass's theory is best rebutted not by challenging his theory of human nature but by challenging the claims he makes about its moral relevance.

Nonetheless, there are glimmers in Kass's writings of a grander vision. He has a tendency, for example, to speak broadly of human nature as a kind of touchstone or guiding light in thinking about biotechnology. *Beyond Therapy,* a report from the President's Council on Bioethics and heavily influenced by Kass, asserts that "only if there is a *human* 'givenness,' or a given humanness, that is also good and worth respecting, . . . will the 'given' serve as a *positive* guide for choosing what to alter and what to leave alone" (2003, p. 289). Also, it is striking that Kass reaches skeptical conclusions about enhancement every time he considers it; though the method is case by case, the underlying agenda is general. If human nature is not a straightforward moral guide, it nonetheless provides something close to a guide. Finally, there is an undercurrent in Kass's writings of essentialism. Kass emphasizes the limits of science and empiricism and the room, and need, for alternative ways of apprehending human life. "Our current evolutionary orthodoxy," he notes, "has, in fact, little to say about the true origin of life or about ultimate causes, not only of life but of all major biological novelty. It cannot account for the emergence of higher organisms" (2004, p. 288). We need to turn, Kass tells us, to "unorthodox biologists," and in particular to Aristotle, "who emphasized questions of being over becoming, form over matter, purposiveness over moving parts, and wholes over parts; for whom the soul was not an ethereal spirit or a ghost-in-the-machine but an immanent and embodied principle of all vital activity; and for whom science was a refined and ever-deepening reflection the natures and causes of the beings manifest to us in ordinary experience" (p. 294).

It is hard to read such passages without concluding that Kass thinks, at some level, that the cosmos is rationally ordered, that humans—highest of the higher organisms—have their proper place in the overall order, and that understanding their nature is, not merely a matter of collecting observations about what humans are like, but also a matter of gaining special insight into larger mysteries (p. 296; Kass emphasizes the importance of mysteries here). These grander ambitions for deploying the concept suggest a commitment to a much stronger theory of human nature than Kass ever attempts to provide.

Human Nature as a Condition of Morality

Another way of thinking about the moral relevance of human nature is to see it as a logical requirement of (human) morality. Francis Fukuyama takes this approach. Fukuyama is also the clearest case of someone opposed to enhancing human nature who rests the argument on an overarching theory of human nature. Fukuyama claims, famously, that human nature "is the sum of the behavior and characteristics that are typical of the human species, arising from genetic rather than environmental factors" (2002, p. 130). Thus, humans are distinguished by an overall set of traits, rather than any one trait; Fukuyama does not attempt a complete list. In fact, the set would have to be somewhat indeterminate, if only because, as noted above, any attempt to specify "fundamental facts" tends to be indeterminate. Further, the set will consist of ranges of traits rather than precisely specified traits. Because traits are a function of environmental as well as genetic factors, the set of traits "arising from genetic factors" will be unstable; "normal human height," for example, can change over the generations due to changes in diet. Nonetheless, out of this overall general understanding of the range of traits possible given the human genome emerges what is distinctively human, which Fukuyama calls "the human essence" or "Factor X." This is not itself a trait but an emergent property that depends on the entirety of human traits. Thus, though Fukuyama holds that human nature is definable, he does not hold that we can easily articulate human nature: "If what gives us dignity and a moral status higher than that of other living creatures is related to the fact that we are complex wholes rather than the sum of simple parts, then it is clear that there is no simple answer to the question, What is Factor X? That is, Factor X cannot be reduced to the possession of moral choice, or reason, or language, or sociability, or sentience, or emotions, or consciousness, or any other quality that has been put forth as a ground for human dignity. It is all of these qualities coming together in a human whole that make up Factor X" (p. 171).

Fukuyama's problem with enhancement technologies is that if we shift human nature beyond the pale of the traits that our genes make possible, then we will disrupt our understanding of human dignity and therefore of human rights.

Given his understanding of "the human essence" as emergent from the overall set of human traits, Fukuyama maintains a broad opposition to enhancement. "What is it we want to protect from any future advances in biotechnology? The answer is, we want to protect the full range of our complex, evolved natures against attempts at self-modification" (p. 172). In other words, it is not only language and rationality but also the entire set of behavioral and physical characteristics that concerns Fukuyama. His opposition is also stringent; the apparent implication is that even relatively small changes—giving humans greater height or strength, for example—might be threatening.

Plainly, this stance toward enhancement requires that we have a pretty good understanding of human nature. The core of the problem is that Fukuyama attaches value primarily to human species norms, with the added complication that he sees norms as established genetically. We have to be able to enumerate the traits we must watch, fix their appropriate ranges, and sort out the genetic contribution to them. But getting a handle on all this—especially sorting out the genetic versus the environmental contributions to traits—has proven difficult. Another part of the problem is Fukuyama's flirtation with essentialism. His broad and stringent set of traits that ought not be genetically modified amounts to an attempt to define decisively what falls into and what outside the human category. But this will give some perplexing results, as Nicholas Agar notes (2004, p. 96). It may imply, for example, that Shaquille O'Neal, whose height is certainly anomalous, is not fully human. Fukuyama is aware of this danger, and he takes pains to emphasize that traits vary greatly and that gene-environment interactions can shift the entire range of traits over time. He allows that "there are doubtless some mutant female kangaroos born without pouches"—kangaroos despite the fact that having pouches is part of "kangarooness" (2002, p. 135). A universal need not literally be universal; "it needs rather to have a single, distinct median or modal point, and a relatively small standard deviation."

However, a latitudinarian approach to hard cases tends to make rigorous opposition to enhancement difficult to sustain. If we allow that a pouchless kangaroo is still a kangaroo and Shaquille O'Neal is still a man, then we might also be able to say that an enhanced human is not, in fact, *post*-human. Enhancement that does not bump a person beyond the range of normality might be unobjectionable, and enhancement that shifts someone outside the range of normality might not *always* make human dignity and human rights inapplicable. Enhancement would seem to pose a problem only when it occurs often enough and dramatically enough to pull apart the statistical curves that describe normal ranges of human traits. It is broad social trends that we are really concerned about, not individuals.

A nonessentialist version of Fukuyama's general approach seems possible. Paul Lauritzen argues that if biotechnology can significantly change human capabilities and life trajectories but is not available to most people, then it risks undermining our common sense of humanity, which could undermine the capacity for human sympathy (2005, p. 28). The starting point for this thought is that human identity is bound up with human biology, such that "a new biology might give rise to a new psychology." A new psychology would lead, in turn, to a new ethics. In particular, worries Lauritzen, it would challenge our conception of human rights. "The most persuasive account of human rights," he writes, "is framed in relation to the notion of a stable human nature." The fear, then, "is that biotechnology will change the species-typical characteristics shared by all humans. If that happens, and if rights are tied to a conception of human nature that is in turn rooted in a biological reality, then biotechnology threatens the very basis of human morality as we know it."

In Lauritzen's view, then, it is critical to human morality that there is a stable human nature and that humans all recognize that there is a stable human morality. But "a stable human nature" does not imply *unique* human nature. Lauritzen is not concerned to show that we can show what is inside and what is outside the human category. His point is only that we must have some ability to describe important human characteristics that people of different races, ethnicities, sexes, and nationalities share in roughly the same measures. We might start the way Nussbaum does, by developing lists of key human capacities, while acknowledging that the lists are always open-ended and contestable. To do so is to speak of human norms, but it is not to make the norm itself the locus of value. In short, Lauritzen is not committed to anything more than an ongoing exploration of human nature.

The Relationship between Humans and Nature

Another way of arguing for the moral significance of human nature is to argue that a certain kind of relationship to it is morally significant. Michael Sandel and Jürgen Habermas exemplify this approach. Sandel argues that a certain relationship to human nature is both valued in itself and vital for various things that we value in human society, and Habermas claims that a certain relationship to human nature is vital for equal membership in the moral community.

Sandel's argument for worrying about enhancement is broad ranging, and in places he seems to develop arguments that follow consequentialist lines. His primary argument, though, is that certain ways of using enhancement lead to an imbalance in two sorts of relationships to human nature—an accepting relationship, in which we see nature as a gift, and a perfectionist relationship, in which we strive to improve it. The ideal is to hold these in tension with each other, but enhancement pushes us away from the first and toward the second. Widespread use of enhancement would "represent the one-sided triumph of willfulness over giftedness, of dominion over reverence, of molding over beholding" (2007, p. 85).

Sandel goes on to say why losing "the ethic of giftedness" would be unfortunate, but these final observations work more to elaborate what is wrong about losing giftedness than to explain it. Losing the ethic of giftedness would undermine "three key features of our moral landscape—humility, responsibility, and solidarity." This claim could be understood as a consequentialist point—if we lose these key constraints on our behavior, many people will end up worse off—or it might be understood as pointing out conceptual implications—if we lose these aspects of the "moral landscape," we could not but feel that as a huge loss. Sandel plainly hopes, though, that many of his readers will feel the loss of giftedness itself already as a loss. It is partly to show the import of losing giftedness itself that he tries to show how it is bound up in sports and in parenthood, such that if we lose the ethic of giftedness, then sports and parenthood will be diminished— "the drive to banish contingency and to master the mystery of birth diminishes the designing parent and corrupts parenting as a social practice governed by norms of unconditional love" (pp. 82–83). Sandel's argument is not limited to sports and parenthood, however; he intends these discussions to exemplify a larger point about giftedness.

For my purposes, the important point is that Sandel can speak of the human relationship to bodily nature without making any overarching claim about human nature itself, other than that the traits people have depend on the bodies they have and that traditionally people have acquired their bodies and therefore their traits through contingent processes rather than through design. The point of giftedness is that we do not know exactly what to expect in human nature, so we should foster an "openness to the unbidden" (a phrase he draws from William May, who served with Sandel on the President's Council on Bioethics). But such claims fall well shy of a theory of human nature.

Contingency is also critical in Habermas's case against enhancement. We are able to live together in communities and engage each other as equals because we all share some sort of "prior ethical self-understanding"—an understanding of who we are that makes it possible for us to see ourselves as "ethically free and

morally equal beings" (2003, pp. 38–41). If I understand Habermas right, the critical element in this self-understanding is an awareness that we are embodied and
that our bodies are our own, in the sense that we do not acquire them from other
people; they are products of fate or nature rather than of other members of
the community. In short, the contingent nature of a person's traits is a condition
of being one's own person—of having autonomy, having unique worth, being a
member of equal standing in the moral community. We must be able to assume
that "we act and judge *in propria persona*—that it is our own voice speaking and
no other" (p. 57).

Habermas worries that this assumption is at risk if a child knows that she has
been genetically enhanced by her parents, for then the parents' goals are present
directly in her body. The processes of child-rearing and socialization may also
impose the parents' goals on the child, but the child can in principle reject these,
and Habermas supposes that such goals will not be present in the child's body in
the same way. Of course, the child might accept her parents' goals as her own,
and if she does, she will not feel deprived of her own voice. But because we cannot be sure that children's and parents' goals will harmonize, genetically enhancing children "jeopardizes a precondition for the moral self-understanding of
autonomous actors" (p. 63). Thus, parents should approach parenthood with an
"expectation of the unexpected" (a phrase Habermas draws from Hannah Ar-
endt; see p. 58).

Whether either Sandel's or Habermas's concerns are ultimately persuasive depends on pursuing moral and political questions that lie beyond the scope of this
chapter. Much more would have to be said to support Habermas's argument, in
particular, because it aims at more than Sandel's, or at least, it aims at more than
Sandel's *need* aim. Sandel's argument can be understood simply as identifying
and defending a personal moral ideal, one that many people share and that Sandel
wants to recommend, but which he would not seek to enforce through public
policy. Habermas, however, must be aiming at public policy. To wrongly prevent
some people from joining the moral community is to commit a grave injustice
that must be opposed by law. Thus, Habermas's argument must meet a higher
burden of proof than Sandel's.

Both positions rest on claims about human nature that are modest and defensible. Neither is making any claims about human beings' essential nature. Nor is
either arguing that a normal human range of traits is what we value. Indeed,
neither identifies any *particular* desirable human traits at all; it is the *relationship*
to human nature that they are concerned about. For each, it is enough to say that

individual human beings come into the world with their own natures; for us to assert (too much) control over others' natures is troublesome.

If I have characterized Habermas's argument correctly, the key point he wants to make about our understanding of human nature is only that we exist in bodies that do not incorporate the intentions of other members of the community. There is no expectation that we have thoroughly catalogued the traits that make up human nature, much less that we have come up with a *definition* of human nature that sets out a criterion for those traits. Further, Habermas's emphasis on contingency does not imply that human nature is fixed. It might indeed change, but the change must itself be contingent. Natural evolution seems acceptable, for example. The constraint Habermas would impose is only on how the change occurs; some members of the community should not be able to deliberately intervene in the bodies of other members.

The complexity of the genes' contribution to actual human life may qualify Habermas's and Sandel's concerns about modifying children. Parents' success at using genetic technologies to *make* their children turn out one way rather than another is likely to vary greatly, depending on what traits they have in mind for their children, and it may well be that a majority of the traits parents would want to produce lie beyond genetic control. It does not take complete success at controlling a trait to raise concerns, however. Completely controlling a trait might be the limit case. Habermas would be troubled if an intervention falls short but leaves a lasting reminder for the child—on the child—of what the parents wanted the child to be (though more needs to be said about whether lasting bodily reminders of parents' plans would affect the child's sense of autonomy). Sandel's worry that the child is not regarded to a sufficient degree as a gift depends on the parents' attitudes, which (Sandel supposes) depend in part on parents' capacity to carry out their own plans. But parents might fail to regard a child as a gift even though they have little or no ability to modify the child's given traits. Plainly, then, both Habermas's and Sandel's concerns are matters of degree. (Sandel is explicit on this score because he is uneasy that the two competing attitudes might shift out of balance.) Worries about parental control of children would grow as parents are able to affect how their children turn out.

If concerns about genetic interventions are explained in terms of parents' attitudes and children's self-understanding, then plainly there is no sharp line demarcating genetic from environmental interventions. To the degree that an environmental change leaves a permanent reminder of the parents' own intentions for the child (consider surgery to Westernize the eyes of an Asian child adopted by

Western parents), it ought to generate both Habermas's and Sandel's concerns every bit as much as it would if accomplished through genetic intervention. The genes are not special repositories of value. The point is rather that the relationship in which we stand to human nature(s), and to the natures of our children, is a matter of human value.

The Relationship between Human Nature and the Human Good

One feature common to Fukuyama, Habermas, and Sandel is that they offer general claims about the undesirability of intervening in human nature. Kass, too, seems to have a general agenda, even though his method of argument seems otherwise. But one might instead tackle the issue of human enhancement in a much more limited way, arguing merely that there are some features of human nature that should not be changed or even that there are contexts in which certain features of human nature should not be changed.

This kind of approach is exemplified by Thomas Murray. Murray suggests that we think of human nature as providing "the contours of the given" and then consider the implications of changing those contours for different social practices. The social import or meaning of some practices depends on having certain complex relationships to the human given, and it can be undermined if it is altered through biotechnological shortcuts. In thinking about sports and parent-child relationships, for example, Murray reaches conclusions similar to Kass's: enhancement in sports is at odds with the very meaning of sports because "what we look for in athletes is a combination of *natural talents* and the *virtuous perfection* of those talents" (2007, p. 513). Athletic competition can be conceived of along different lines, Murray observes, but then the meaning of the practice is different, sufficiently different that those competitions seem distinguishable from sports proper. Maximum performance, instead of natural talents honed through hard work, becomes the object. Similarly, parental enhancement is at odds with the values that shape the parent-child relationship. Parents should accept their children "as they are, with their appetites and enthusiasms, fears and aspirations, however that personal reality might diverge from our idealized image of the child we dreamt of having" (p. 508). But Murray concludes that enhancement need not always be opposed; in some cases, what is plainly enhancement would even be desirable. If surgeons could take pills that steadied their hands or allowed them to remain alert through long surgeries, they probably should do it (p. 503).

Murray, too, is not committed to an overall theory of human nature. His claim is not that human nature in general is valuable but that, in some contexts, we have reason to value human nature as we find it. If we are opposed to sports doping, for example, then we will be concerned about aspects of human nature relevant to that sport, as that sport is understood. Sports often incorporate or permit a certain amount of enhancement; bicycles and tennis rackets are sometimes said to be mechanical enhancements of a sort. That's fine. The bicycling enthusiast need not have thought that all human enhancement is wrong, but only that given the way the sport of bicycling is constituted and instituted, *this array* of human enhancements are undesirable.

Another version of this limited approach to thinking about human enhancement would be to make general, non-context-dependent claims about specific aspects of human nature, again without being committed to a complete account of human nature. The philosophical movement known as "transhumanism" helps elaborate this point. As the name suggests, transhumanism tacitly rests on some understanding of human nature. Rather than valuing that nature, however, transhumanists see it as a condition that we should strive to transcend. We should rid ourselves of the animal portion of our nature. We should be much smarter than we are, much longer lived and ideally immortal, able to cognize without being grounded by emotions, and able to craft our lives without being limited by an instinct to affiliate with other people. If we were largely cut loose from our bodies, we might also have different views about sexuality and music. Transhumanists would retain (and refine) other aspects of human nature, especially the capacity to set goals and deliberate about how best to pursue them (Agar, 2007). But while they have some particular ideas about how we should get better, they need not have a complete account either of what we are or of the species we are to become. Exactly what we would turn out to value, once we reached our new state, might be entirely impossible for us to say in our present limited state.

Conversely, what we might think of as a "mere humanist" might value an assortment of things about being human—items from Arnhart's and Nussbaum's lists, for example—without having a definitive or exhaustive account of what a human being is. (If we set aside Kass's grander aspirations to an understanding of human nature beyond what observation alone can provide, this limited approach might be his method. As it is, though, perhaps we should label Kass a "transcendental humanist.") The mere humanist can allow that there is no account that ties together, conceptually, every item on a particular list of human nature, and she can acknowledge that the list itself is open-ended and contestable. The fifth item on Nussbaum's list is "emotions": "Being able to have attachments to things and people outside ourselves; to love those who love and care for us, to

grieve at their absence; in general, to love, to grieve, to experience longing, gratitude, and justified anger" (2006, p. 79). Having emotions is a feature of our ani-
mality, and perhaps something we might, in some bizarre future world, be able to
greatly diminish or move beyond. But it does seem to be a feature of human life
that a humanist would value.

Statements about the value of humanity tend to blend at this point with statements about "human flourishing." Nussbaum holds that the ten capacities she
identifies are the minimal conditions for a life with human dignity. In a marvel-
ous set of essays on the breadth of parents' freedom to choose the kind of children
they wish to have, Jonathan Glover seems at one point to set to one side concerns
about the intrinsic value of human nature: "In the early days of the debate on genetic enhancement, some of the objections raised (such as that it would be 'unnatural') were based mainly on emotional revulsion ('the yu[c]k factor'). Some
people still have this kind of revulsion. But one result of twenty years' discussion
is that these responses have been questioned and largely put aside. Now the serious debate is in the spirit of the harm principle and reflects concern for people.
The impact of genetic enhancement on human flourishing, on the kinds of lives
people will lead, is central" (2006, p. 76).

In the closing section of the book, however, Glover contemplates whether parents' choices may need some sort of restraint, and he considers several possible
bases for these restraints—to prevent social inequalities, to keep parents from
falling into self-defeating competitions, to protect the child's right to an open
future. "And, perhaps most fundamentally, the limits may be needed to protect
parts of human nature needed either for the containment of our dark side *or else
in a more positive way for the good life, parts of our nature that it would be tragic
to lose*" (p. 103, emphasis added).

Glover has reason to say that *losing valuable parts of our nature* raises a concern about human flourishing rather than human nature. Perhaps concerns
about human flourishing are less likely to be blanket judgments than are claims
about human nature. Perhaps it encourages a more considered moral position
because we recognize the necessity of weighing different ways of flourishing.
(What's objectionable about "the yuck factor" is its seeming thoughtlessness.) But
if there is some feature of human existence that we not only value now but also
would prefer future generations valued—the presence in human life of emotions,
sociability, limits to parental control over children, sexuality, or something more
specific such as humor or love of music—then we are saying something more than
that we value human flourishing. We are saying that we value a rich conception

of human flourishing that includes some of the traditional forms that seem to be part of human nature as it has existed until now. We are then making a de facto appeal to human nature.

The Politics of "Human Nature"

Many arguments about the biotechnological alteration of human nature do not make grand claims about human nature. The meaningful objections to these arguments are not to the concept of human nature but to the moral value attached to it—that they are not constitutive of human dignity, that they are not necessary for the special goods found in certain human practices, that a certain relationship to nature has no particular moral significance, or that human nature is not bound up with key moral values (let alone with morality in general).

One might also ask questions about the significance of whatever moral value is attached to human nature. These questions shift the focus from the first to the last half of the quick and crude objection: "X is against nature, and therefore wrong." If X is *wrong,* then it might be publicly enforceable, and perhaps some people fear that moral concerns about human nature will lead to policies that restrict individual liberty in ways they find objectionable. This is a question both of political and moral philosophy.

Government policy must rest on reasons that are accessible to and assessable by the public; it must be possible for the governed to see why a policy has been enacted and to independently evaluate that explanation. Further, government policy must rest on moral positions that achieve some threshold of general acceptance. In Rawls's formulation, those positions must be part of an "overlapping consensus" of the many different "comprehensive world views" that may be held in a liberal democracy. Given these requirements, a government policy could not rest on claims about human nature unless those claims could be well defended. Essentialist conceptions of human nature would be ruled out from the start. Other claims about human nature might be ruled out because they are factually wrong. (Government policy on education, family, and health is subject to the same sorts of restrictions.) Yet other positions might not pass muster not because they make claims about the moral significance of human nature that are not sufficiently widely shared.

Moral views about human nature, even if widely shared, might not be the kind of thing we think suitable for legal enforcement. Perhaps the moral attitude toward human nature is a kind of *ideal* one holds for the relationship between humans and nature. It might be similar in ways to some ideals we have for relationships between humans, such as that a person tends to treat others with warmth or generosity. Such an ideal would not issue in blunt pronouncements that something is right or wrong, permissible or impermissible. For a person who holds it, it would be action-guiding, and that person might think better of other people who demonstrate it—indeed, we might still think it an important feature of the moral life—but at the same time, we would not expect everybody to have it, and we would stop well short of thinking that people who lack it are to that degree *immoral*. They just do not live up to a standard we set for ourselves.

Perhaps, too, this gives one final reason that one need not have a full theory of human nature to have moral qualms about altering it. If a liberty-restricting government policy on, say, research into human cloning rests on claims about human nature, then the requirement that those claims be publicly accessible and assessable raises the bar for whatever we might claim about human nature. A publicly enforceable moral standard would require a convergence of opinion about human nature, a collective weighing and sifting. A personal moral standard can be based on one's own considered assessments, and perhaps even on one's own best guesses.

NOTES

1. I am thinking here of a variety of conversations and conferences I have found myself part of, rather than of any particular critic's published material. Pointing this out may make the position look like a straw man, but I have now heard it often enough, in enough different venues, to believe that many critics see moral concerns of human nature as boiling down to a position along these lines.

2. Yet another line of defense would be to note the limitations of any moral ideal about the intrinsic value of human nature: concerns about nature are often far from decisive either morally or politically.

3. See, for example, Kittay, who expresses this thought by saying that we "normalize the anomalous" (2006, p. 100).

REFERENCES

Agar, N. 2004. *Liberal Eugenics: In Defence of Human Enhancement*. Oxford: Blackwell.
———. 2007. "Whereto Transhumanism? The Literature Reaches a Critical Mass." *Hastings Center Report* 37 (4): 12–17

Arnhart, L. 1998. *Darwinian Natural Right: The Biological Ethics of Human Nature.* Albany, N.Y.: State University of New York Press.

Asch, A. 2006. "Appearance-Altering Surgery, Children's Sense of Self, and Parental Love." In *Surgically Shaping Children: Technology, Ethics, and the Pursuit of Normality,* ed. E. Parens, pp. 227–52. Baltimore: Johns Hopkins University Press.

Ehrlich, P. 2000. *Human Natures: Genes, Cultures, and the Human Prospect.* New York: Penguin.

Fukuyama, F. 2002. *Our Posthuman Future: Consequences of the Biotechnology Revolution.* New York: Farrar, Straus & Giroux.

Glover, J. 2006. *Choosing Children: Genes, Disability, and Design.* New York: Oxford University Press.

Habermas, J. 2003. *The Future of Human Nature.* Cambridge, U.K.: Polity Press, in association with Blackwell.

Kass, L. R. 2004. *Life, Liberty, and the Defense of Dignity: The Challenge for Bioethics.* San Francisco: Encounter Books.

Kittay, E. 2006. "Thoughts on the Desire for Normality." In *Surgically Shaping Children: Technology, Ethics, and the Pursuit of Normality,* ed. E. Parens, pp. 99–110. Baltimore: Johns Hopkins University Press.

Lauritzen, P. 2005. "Stem Cells, Biotechnology, and Human Rights: Implications for a Posthuman Future." *Hastings Center Report* 35 (2): 25–33.

Midgley, M. 1979. *Beast and Man: The Roots of Human Nature.* London: Routledge.

Mill, J. S. 1961. "On Nature." In *Essential Works of John Stuart Mill,* ed. M. Lerner, pp. 367–401. New York: Bantam.

Murray, T. H. 2007. "Enhancement." In *The Oxford Handbook of Bioethics,* ed. B. Steinbock, pp. 491–515. New York: Oxford University Press.

Nussbaum, M. 2000. *Women and Human Development: The Capabilities Approach.* Cambridge, U.K.: Cambridge University Press.

———. 2006. *Frontiers of Justice: Disability, Nationality, Species Membership.* Cambridge, Mass.: Belknap Press of Harvard University Press.

President's Council on Bioethics. 2003. *Beyond Therapy: Biotechnology and the Pursuit of Happiness.* Washington, D.C.

Sandel, M. 2007. *The Case against Perfection: Ethics in the Age of Genetic Engineering.* Cambridge, Mass.: Belknap Press of Harvard University Press.

CHAPTER FIVE

Preserving the Distinction between Nature and Artifact

Eric Katz, Ph.D.

Is "nature" a significant moral category for the development of public policy? The answer to this question depends on what public policy is being considered. The utility of the concept of nature for ethical and policy decisions cannot be determined universally and a priori; rather, it exists along a spectrum of relevance and appropriateness, and it must be determined pragmatically based on the specific facts of each individual situation. In the area of environmental policy, for example, the idea of nature—indeed, nature's actual existence as a physical reality—plays an important role in determining the ethical basis of policy decisions. Nonetheless, the idea of nature is not always of prime importance in environmental policy, for when we consider environmental issues in largely artifactual realms, such as urban centers, the idea of what is natural is little help in determining appropriate policy decisions. In human health and medical policy, as another example, the concept of nature plays a much less important role. Yet the spectrum of relevance exists in this area also, for some medical decisions are based on an idea of what is natural for the human body, even though most medical procedures seek to interfere with or modify the natural processes of disease, injury, or deterioration.

Is there a key—a rubric, principle, or algorithm—for understanding the application of this spectrum of relevance regarding the use of nature in policy decisions? I believe that there is such a key and that it concerns the distinction between naturally occurring entities and human-created artifactual products, or more simply, between *nature* and *artifacts*. By *nature,* I mean the realm of entities and processes unmodified by human agency; I consider the world of *artifacts* to be the realm in which entities and processes are modified and created by human intention and human manipulation. The role of the concept of nature in policy decisions thus rests primarily on the extent to which the decision concerns either the natural realm or the human or artifactual realm. If we are to employ the concept of nature in policy-making decisions, then we must maintain the distinction between *nature* and *artifacts*—on one side, the unmodified natural processes of the world that denote the world of nature and, on the other side, the results and products of human intentionality and manipulation of those processes that tend to create an artifactual human world.

In this chapter I argue that the preservation of the distinction between nature and artifacts is a crucial feature of our analysis of the ethics of policy decisions. This analysis involves a two-step process.[1] First, we must understand the real ontological difference between natural entities and artifacts. Second, we must recognize the normative value of the distinction. I use my previous work in the ethics of the policy of ecological restoration as the primary focus of this argument, but I also extend the discussion into areas involving human medical practice, broadly conceived as the attempt to modify natural processes in the development of human organisms. My conclusion is that there is a moral reason for preserving the distinction between nature and artifacts. The moral significance of this distinction rests on the concepts of intervention and domination.

The Nature/Artifact Distinction: Restoration and Its Meaning

In a series of articles I began publishing around 1991, I argued that ecological restorations (and to a certain extent, policies of natural resource management) do not actually restore or manage "natural systems."[2] I concluded that the restoration and re-creation of damaged natural environments is a misdirection in environmental policy, the result of a misunderstanding of the human role in shaping and determining environmental processes.

What is ecological restoration? It is a scientific and technological enterprise, geared to the restoration, repair, and re-creation of natural ecosystems and landscapes. At one extreme, it is the mitigation of systems damaged by human interference, such as the cleaning up of the Exxon Valdez oil spill. At another extreme, it is an attempt to "cover up," literally, an intentional disruption of natural areas, such as the re-creation and replanting of a mountainside after strip-mining for coal. There is also a vast array of middle positions, such as the attempt to re-create historical landscapes or ecosystems that no longer exist for the purpose of extracting scientific knowledge. Steve Packard's attempt to re-create the oak-savannah plains of the U.S. Midwest is an early and prominent example of one of these middle positions (Packard, 1988).

Why would I criticize the repair of damaged ecosystems or the re-creation of historic landscapes? Begin with the terminology: the idea that human technology and science can restore a natural environment is a perversion of the word *restore*. We cannot *restore* a natural environment; at best we can create a perfect substitute, but this substitute is an artifact created by human beings, not a naturally occurring entity or system. It is a product of human intention and design.

Consider this process in more detail: once a system has been created, designed, or managed by human technology and science, it is no longer a natural system; it is now an artifact, a product of human intention and design. There is a fundamental ontological difference in the essential character of natural entities and human artifacts. Artifacts exist only because of human intention and design. Artifacts are the physical manifestation of human purpose imposed on the world of nature. An artifact would not be conceived, designed, or created unless it was thought to promote some human purpose. *This is completely unlike the origin of natural entities.* Natural entities, of course, do not exist through any process of design or purpose—unless we want to ignore post-Darwinian science and raise a whole host of theological questions, which I think it is better to avoid. (But note that even if we consider the natural world to have been designed by God, it would still be fundamentally different from a world created by human design for human purposes. We cannot assume that God designed the world for human good, or that God's intentionality is similar to human intentionality.) Once we inject our intentional designs into a natural system, we no longer have a natural system; we have a garden, a forest plantation, or a farm. We may create a landscape that appears to be a natural wilderness because for various reasons we appreciate the look and experience of wilderness, but this wilderness is a human-made artifact that merely resembles the wilderness produced by natural processes.

Based on the fundamental difference between artifacts and naturally occurring entities, I questioned the meaning of ecological restoration and the policies of sustainable forestry, and I used the provocative phrase "the big lie" to characterize the policy of the "restoration of nature." Once we see that the introduction of human intentionality and purpose fundamentally changes the character of a natural system, then we cannot say that we are restoring nature. Instead, we are creating artifactual systems—or, at best, hybrid systems of natural entities and artifacts—that are designed to achieve some set of human purposes or benefits. These human benefits may be significant and important, and thus the policies of restoration and management may be justified in particular cases, but they should not be characterized as the restoration of nature. The danger in misunderstanding the meaning of these environmental polices is an increased "humanization" of the natural world, the limitless expansion of human power to mold and manipulate the natural world. The specter of domination as the fundamental policy of human activity begins to haunt us.

Let me consider two objections to this analysis. The late Richard Sylvan argued that my idea of an artifact as applied to natural systems was too expansive, too broad. For Sylvan (1994), not all restorations are artifactual because nature can heal itself. In time, nature can wash out human influence. As an example, consider the case of a garden that needs to be tended and maintained by continuous human action and intervention; if the human maintenance activity is ended, nature will reassert itself, and in time the garden will become wild again. Now it is true that without continuous human interventions nature will prevail in the future development of environmental and biological systems, but the fact remains that the progress of the natural system will be different after the initial human intervention. The resulting system will be different from what would have been the case had no intervention taken place at all. Following Sylvan, we might not want to call the resulting system an artifact because it is no longer guided by human intentionality and purpose, yet the system is not equivalent to undisturbed nature. Indeed, placing our hopes on the power of nature to heal itself does not eliminate the danger of human domination of natural systems. The belief that nature is so powerful that it can heal itself no matter what humans do to it is the mirror image of the belief that humanity can control, heal, and restore the natural world. The belief in an omnipotent nature correcting our mistakes is simply a moral rationalization of the human desire to control natural processes for the furtherance of human interests.

It may also be objected that my position reinforces both a conceptual and an ontological dualism between humanity and nature or, more precisely, between culture and nature. I accept this characterization of my position; it is dualistic. But I do not consider this dualism to be pernicious or a reason that my analysis is incorrect. The often-quoted mantra of the environmental movement that "humans are a part of nature" is a prime example of fuzzy thinking. Of course, humans are biological beings, and thus in some sense natural, but we humans have lived for the last ten thousand years (at least) as cultural beings, modifying natural processes to suit our needs and interests. We live our lives in a cultural world, what Jacques Ellul called a technological milieu; we do not live in nature.

But the dualism of artifacts and natural entities is not absolute. Naturalness and artifactuality exist along a spectrum of various kinds of entities. Things can be more or less natural, more or less artifactual. A wooden chair is more natural than a plastic chair because it is more closely related to the naturally produced material that forms its basic structure. The plastic chair is farther from its original material or source. But both chairs are definitely artifacts, essentially different from naturally occurring entities, a fallen tree that I sit on while walking through the forest, for example. Why are the chairs different from the fallen tree? Because they are the result of human intention, human design, and the human manipulation of natural materials and processes. We could stand around forever and watch nonhuman nature at work and we will *never* see it produce a chair. Although human beings are biological beings, the products of an evolutionary process, what we humans do—the things we create, build, make, imagine—these are all artifactual, with a source outside the realm of naturally occurring entities, processes, and systems. Our artifacts, our culture, would not exist if we humans had not intentionally interfered with and molded the natural world. Nature alone could not create the world in which we now find ourselves.

Consider a series of cases that I wrote about in a previous essay (Katz, 2000, pp. 41–42). These cases illustrate the difference between natural changes in a system and human-induced artifactual changes, and they also show that the differences between artifacts and natural entities are relative, existing along a spectrum. The cases concern the reintroduction of wolves into Yellowstone National Park, a designated wilderness area. Is the reintroduction of wolves into Yellowstone the restoration of nature? Consider a range of cases, some true, some merely possible:

1. Wild wolves, never captured or bred by humans, migrate on their own from Canada into Yellowstone and establish several distinct packs in different regions of the park.
2. Some wild Canadian wolves are captured by U.S. scientists and released into Yellowstone, where they establish several distinct packs in different regions of the park.

3. Some Canadian wolves are captured by U.S. scientists, bred extensively in captivity, and then released into Yellowstone, where they establish several distinct packs in different regions of the park.
4. Good wolf specimens from several zoological parks are bred together and the offspring released into Yellowstone, where they establish several distinct packs in different regions of the park.
5. Using the most recent genetic engineering techniques, several wolves are cloned, then bred in captivity, and their offspring are released into Yellowstone, where they establish several distinct packs in different regions of the park.

Now imagine that "on the ground," the ecological consequences of all five cases are indistinguishable. All five cases lead to the flourishing of wolves in the wilderness area, and thus the reintroduction of natural predation—a result that all environmentalists (of a preservationist bent) would find satisfactory. But are all the cases the same? Are they of equal value? I would argue that the essential characters of the cases are not similar; the cases exhibit an ontological difference.

So what is actually going on when we do ecological restoration? We are creating artifactual systems that resemble nature, but they are not an authentic nature because of the presence of human intentionality (and human technology and science). This does not make restoration an evil policy of action. Clearly, ecological restoration, when it is a policy advocated by committed environmentalists, is a policy designed to improve the world. But its fundamental ontological meaning ought to give us pause.

We can now move on to the second step of the process. Because we have established the ontological difference between nature and artifacts, we must examine the normative value of the distinction. One obvious, but incorrect, method of assigning normative value here would be to assume that the dualism of ontological meaning is matched by a dualism of normative value, so that, for example, natural entities are considered "good" while artifactual entities are considered "evil," or vice versa. This kind of oversimplification, which we sometimes see in advertisements for "green" or "natural" consumer products (such as organic dry cleaning) or in arguments for medical interventions (such as Lasik surgery to improve natural vision), is clearly inadequate for an understanding of the complex array of values present in natural entities and artifactual products. A simple dualism will not provide us with the correct algorithm needed to assign the proper normative values.

Returning to an analysis of the policy of restoration may offer direction. As I have demonstrated, the policy of restoration is an activity that creates a system of artifacts. It is a policy based on the assumption that artifacts created by human intention and design will significantly improve the state of the world. Simply put, human activity creates a better world. The human modification of natural processes produces positive value. Surely, this is the fundamental assumption of the human engagement with the natural world: we act to make the world better. Whether we are dealing with the birth of agriculture to insure a continuous food supply or the creation of highways to insure easy transportation or the harnessing of waterways or the atom to produce energy (or hundreds, if not thousands, of other examples), we humans produce goodness.

Ecological restoration, thus, is merely one of the activities or policies that humans use to increase the positive value of the world. It should therefore be a source of positive normative value. Why then do I see restoration as a normative problem? The basic reason is this: it destroys the idea that there is a limit to human action; it assumes that there is a positive value in human omnipotence. Despite its good intentions, the policy of ecological restoration is a manifestation of human hubris. The policy feeds into the human belief—arrogance, really—that we are able to control anything and everything in the natural world. Obviously, this hubris is a trait of human consciousness and human societies and institutions that is as old as civilization itself; that's why the ancient Greeks spent so much time on the subject, and gave us the word itself. I will not, here, make a general argument that acting out of hubris is a poor moral choice; I will assume that we have learned our lesson from a study of the ancient Greek texts, as well as more recent historical examples, that hubris rarely if ever leads to an increase in normative value.

But the specific arrogance of ecological restoration must be noted, as this will aid in our analysis of the value of the nature/artifact distinction. Here the problem is the belief that human science and technology is adequate to create a functioning substitute of a natural system. The activity of restoration requires a functionally equivalent artifactual substitute for the natural system being restored or replaced. Is such a substitute possible? I would like to think that those closest to the field—the ecological restorationists themselves—would realize the futility of trying to re-create natural processes. There is just too much going on within a natural system for us to try to duplicate it through our science and technology. Our knowledge of natural processes is incomplete, and our technological abilities too limited to accomplish the task of restoration. Only an arrogant or hubristic belief in human omnipotence can possibly lead one to think otherwise.

But what if human science and technology were adequate for the policy of restoration? Hypothetically, what if we could know the precise methods of operation of natural processes, and what if we were able to develop technologies that could duplicate nature? Would it then be morally justifiable to pursue ecological restoration as a policy? This is the very situation that Robert Elliot considered when he first introduced the philosophical problem of restoration (1982).[3] Elliot was concerned that developers and despoilers of nature—for example, a strip-mining operation—could use the existence of the science and technology of ecological restoration as an argument to continue to despoil nature. Why not strip mine the mountain if we can restore it to its natural state after we have harvested the coal? Is there an argument that can refute the developer and despoiler of nature? Or do we rest the case for the preservation of nature merely on the empirical fact that we cannot yet completely duplicate natural processes by our restoration science and technology?

This is the crucial issue: restoration ecology is a continuation of the paradigm of human scientific and technological mastery over natural processes. The underlying technological assumption is that humans can control natural processes to better effect than nature can. This assumption changes the nature of environmental policy, moving it away from preservation and protection and replacing it with manipulation and control. The argument will be that anything can be done to a natural entity or system because the despoiled entity or system can be restored later. The concept of preservation will lose all substantive content. It will be a meaningless term in a world of unlimited modification of natural processes.

The ethical or normative conclusion is that human activity regarding the natural environment will know no limits. Humans will manipulate and modify the environment in whatever ways please us. The natural world will have no value except for its usefulness to human projects of control and domination. The world of artifacts will suffice. The idea of human omnipotence regarding the structure and direction of all life will reign supreme. And belief in our omnipotence (and our good intentions and goals) can easily lead to policies of actions that are disastrous in practice and horrible in normative value. Thus it is a moral imperative to maintain the distinction between natural entities and human artifacts. Maintaining this distinction serves as a check on the arrogant notion that human power and human knowledge is unlimited, that human science and technology is capable of dominating and controlling the entire world.

An Extreme Human Case: Nazis and Domination

Can we transfer this analysis of the nature/artifact distinction into the realm of policies of action regarding human beings? The belief in human omnipotence regarding the control of natural processes for the pursuit of human goods may carry over into the realm of strictly human affairs. If the key normative idea is the belief in human omnipotence in the domination and control of natural processes for human good, then we will discover a disturbing parallel situation in the Nazi medical experiments at Auschwitz. The history of the Nazi medical experiments there demonstrates the moral evil of the process of domination, whether this domination applies to humans or to natural processes.[4] Even more strongly, perhaps, we can see that what was wrong with the Nazi medical experiments was primarily the desire to dominate and alter the natural processes involved in the development of humanity.

Consider the experiments of the medical doctor on the notorious Block 10 in Auschwitz, Professor Carl Clauberg. Clauberg injected a caustic substance, now believed to be a combination of Formalin and Novocain, into the cervixes of several hundred women between the ages of twenty and forty. The substance would create adhesions in the fallopian tubes that would cause them to be obstructed. Three to five extremely painful injections were required. The purpose of the experiments was to find a cheap and fast nonsurgical method for sterilizing people thought to be undesirable candidates for reproduction. This would help further the Nazi program of a negative population policy for those thought to be inferior human beings in order to create a biologically pure and healthy race.

Clauberg was not some psychopathic quack or some aberrational Nazi monster dressed in a medical lab coat. On the contrary, according to Robert Jay Lifton, Clauberg was a researcher of high renown. Before the war, he had developed hormonal preparations to treat infertility that are still in use today; he also developed the so-called Clauberg test for measuring the action of progesterone, also still in use today. So in Clauberg we have an example of a leading scientist using the best scientific and technological knowledge available to him to pursue ideological goals that he truly believed were beneficial for society as a whole. That his goals are now considered to be evil is beside the point; what is important here is that science and technology are used to control natural processes, to bend and to manipulate these processes to achieve what are perceived (by the practitioners) as human goods.

The Clauberg case, of course, is not unique among Nazi medical experiments. Consider Josef Mengele's studies of twins, designed to increase the fertility of the German race, or Horst Schumann's experiments in X-ray castration of male prisoners in Birkenau, designed to achieve nonsurgical sterilization in the male population. Other Nazi medical policies included the T-4 euthanasia program for "incurable" medical patients that preceded the "final solution" of the Jewish question and served as its dry run. The point here is not to claim a direct parallel between Nazi medical research and the process of ecological restoration. Rather, the point is that in all of these cases we have examples of the human desire to manipulate, and if need be, distort, natural processes. We have an idea of the arrogance of human power to control the entire dimension of life.

I use the Nazi example purposely (and provocatively) as an extreme instance of human hubris regarding the control of the natural world. If we were to develop a spectrum of the "domination of nature and life-forms, including humans" and index the spectrum with a scale of good to evil, clearly the Nazi medical experiments would lie near the extreme evil side and ecological restoration would be toward the benign end. But the point is that they would both be on the spectrum someplace, for they share one basic, common characteristic: the domination and control of natural processes.

Indeed, the restoration, control, and domination of nature are so explicit in the history and development of Nazism that any environmentalist who supports the management and control of natural ecosystems should feel uncomfortable. It was part of Nazi ideology to remake the world into an Aryan agricultural and Arcadian paradise. Consider the work of architectural historian Robert-Jan Van Pelt, who argues that the reconstruction and redevelopment of Polish farmland under scientific principles of management was one of the major goals of German settlement in the conquered lands east of Germany. Van Pelt writes of a trip by Himmler and his friend Henns Johst, during which they stood in a Polish field, holding the soil in their hands, and dreamed of re-creating German farms and villages; replanting trees, shrubs, and hedgerows; and even altering the climate by increasing dew and the formation of clouds. The goal was a grand re-creation of an organic homeland of blood and soil with a purified Aryan race reigning supreme (1994, pp. 101–3). No better example exists of the ideal of the human domination and control of nature and humanity.

Domination and control are pervasive in any analysis or examination of the policies of the Nazi regime. Consider this memorable passage from Primo Levi, a Holocaust survivor who wrote several books about his imprisonment and survival in the death camps. He writes about the symbolic meanings of three baths that marked his passage from the control of one group to another, the "black-mass bath . . . that marked [the] descent into the concentration camp universe," the "functional, antiseptic" bath of the Americans, and the Russian bath "to human measure, extemporaneous and crude." Of all three baths, he writes, "At each of those three memorable christenings, it was easy to perceive behind the concrete and literal aspect a great symbolic shadow, the unconscious desire of the new authorities, who absorbed us in turn within their own sphere, to strip us of the vestiges of our former life, to make of us new men consistent with their own models, to impose their brand upon us" (1987, p. 8).

Levi's analysis of the meanings of these three baths is a powerful and evocative summary of the human project to control the world and all that lies therein. Evil or benign, the policy of humanity is to dominate, to mold, and to manipulate the raw material presented by nature, to create models of life consistent with the dominant worldview. The Nazi examples illustrate the dangers in the belief that humanity (or a particular subset of humanity) has the power (and the goodwill) to mold the future of all life on earth.

Back to the Nature/Artifact Distinction

Domination, intervention, and control: these are the key concepts to be used in an analysis of the idea of nature as a moral category for the determination of policy. When considering either environmental policy or health policy, we need to examine the extent to which human power is being used to dominate and control all the future developments of the natural world. We need to examine the extent to which we are replacing the world of nature with the realm of artifacts.

My fear is that we will awake one day, in the not too distant future, to a world that is totally artifactual, a fully humanized world without any trace of a spontaneous nonhuman nature that is free to develop according to its own laws. This will be a world of parks, but not of wilderness. It will be a world of playing fields, but not of meadows; a world of canals and waterways, but not of rivers. In the realm of medical policy, it may be a world of designer babies with preselected traits, a world (perhaps) of humans with implanted computer chips to increase memory and the speed of calculation. Considered from the perspective of human life and human accomplishments, this world will not appear to be an evil world at all. Free of disease and pollution, maximizing efficiency in energy and economics, producing a cornucopia of information, foodstuffs, art, science, and various other human pleasures and experiences, this new technological world will produce astonishing amounts of human good and human value. But this new world comes with a cost—a cost, I believe, that is understood only once we see how the dangers of ecological restoration can be universalized into the human realm. The belief that we can intervene, manipulate, and dominate the natural world will produce a starkly different world than the world of nature that surrounds us now. The artifactual world will be a world without nature. It will be a world where human power, science, and technology are able to dominate all natural and all human processes. To prevent this domination and control, to preserve what remains of nature and its spontaneity, it is thus imperative that we maintain the idea that there is a distinction between the natural and the artifactual and use the distinction as a check on the limitless power of humanity to dominate the entire natural and human world.

NOTES

1. Thanks to William Galston for reminding me to make this explicit.

2. See Katz (1992a, 1992b, 1993, 1995). A slightly modified version of "The Big Lie" was published as "Restoration and Redesign: The Ethical Significance of Human Intervention in Nature" (1991). Although this version has an earlier publication date, it actually appeared after the original version of "The Big Lie." These four essays on the ethics of restoration are reprinted in Katz (1997, pp. 93–146). See also Katz (1996, 2000).

3. Elliot expanded his argument into a book: *Faking Nature: The Ethics of Environmental Restoration* (1997). See my critical review of the book in Katz (1998).

4. All the facts cited about the Nazi medical experiments are derived from the classic study by Robert Jay Lifton, *The Nazi Doctors: Medical Killing and the Psychology of Genocide* (1986). For the Clauberg experiments, see pp. 271–78.

REFERENCES

Elliot, R. 1982. "Faking Nature." *Inquiry* 25:81–93.
———. 1997. *Faking Nature: The Ethics of Environmental Restoration*. London: Routledge.
Katz, E. 1991. "Restoration and Redesign: The Ethical Significance of Human Intervention in Nature." *Restoration and Management Notes* 9 (2): 90–96.
———. 1992a. "The Big Lie: Human Restoration of Nature." *Research in Philosophy and Technology* 12:231–41.
———. 1992b. "The Call of the Wild: The Struggle against Domination and the Technological Fix of Nature." *Environmental Ethics* 14:265–73.

———. 1993. "Artifacts and Functions: A Note on the Value of Nature." *Environmental Values* 2:223–32.

———. 1995. "Imperialism and Environmentalism." *Social Theory and Practice* 21 (2): 271–85.

———. 1996. "The Problem of Ecological Restoration." *Environmental Ethics* 18:222–24.

———. 1997. *Nature as Subject: Human Obligation and Natural Community.* Lanham, Md.: Rowman & Littlefield.

———. 1998. Review of Robert Elliot, *Faking Nature: The Ethics of Environmental Restoration. Ethics and the Environment* 3:201–5.

———. 2000. "Another Look at Restoration: Technology and Artificial Nature." In *Restoring Nature: Perspectives from the Social Sciences and Humanities,* ed. P. H. Gobster and R. B. Hull, pp. 37–48. Washington D.C.: Island Press.

Levi, P. 1987. *The Reawakening.* Trans. Stuart Woolf. New York: Collier.

Lifton, R. J. 1986. *The Nazi Doctors: Medical Killing and the Psychology of Genocide.* New York: Basic Books.

Packard, S. 1988. "Just a Few Oddball Species: Restoration and Rediscovery of the Tallgrass Savanna." *Restoration and Management Notes* 6 (1): 13–22.

Sylvan, R. 1994. "Mucking with Nature." In *Against the Mainstream: Critical Environmental Essays,* pp. 48–78. Canberra: Research School of Social Sciences, Australian National University.

Van Pelt, R.-J. 1994. "A Site in Search of a Mission." In *Anatomy of the Auschwitz Death Camp,* ed. Yisrael Gutman and Michael Berenbaum, pp. 93–156. Bloomington: Indiana University Press.

CHAPTER SIX

Why "Nature" Has No Place in Environmental Philosophy

Steven Vogel, Ph.D.

Environmentalism, both as theory and as practice, is traditionally concerned above all with *nature*. Its focus is on protecting nature against the harms generated by human action. The "environment" it wishes to defend is not the built environment of cities, or the technological infrastructure modernity seems to require—although many of us live in urban environments, and the technologies of modernity might be said in a deeper sense to "environ" us all. It is not the nuclear power plants and toxic waste dumps and gridlocked highways surrounding us that environmentalism wants to protect but rather the *natural* environment—an environment that these things instead are said to threaten. Environmental protection means the protection *of nature,* and environmental damage means damage *to nature.* The destruction of something built by humans, like a skyscraper or a dam, does not by itself count as environmental damage. Of course, such destruction may itself have harmful environmental *consequences,* but this only means consequences that are harmful to nature.

Environmental philosophy reflects this concern. Its central theme is to find an appropriate way to understand and defend the ontological and ethical status of nature. Environmental ethicists who want to expand the reach of moral considerability beyond its traditional limitation to humans speak of the "rights of nature"; they do not, typically, worry about the rights of bridges or of toasters. The "environment" spoken of by environmental philosophers is the natural environment;

the built environment—despite the fact that most of us actually live in it—is not usually part of their concern.

Yet to be concerned with the protection of nature, under conditions of modern technological development, is inevitably to worry that it might be too late—that nature might already have ended. This was the famous thesis of Bill McKibben's 1989 book *The End of Nature*. The real core of the "environmental" crisis, McKibben claimed, was that nature itself had literally been destroyed. Particularly as the result of large-scale climate changes produced by human technologies, he suggested, we have entered a new historical stage where no square inch of earth can any longer be called "natural." Human intervention has affected *everything*, and so everything in the world is different from what it would otherwise, "naturally," be. No place is natural any longer, every place is artificial, and so the entire environment has become in a certain sense a built environment. "We have changed the atmosphere and so we are changing the weather," McKibben wrote. "By changing the weather, we make every spot on earth man-made and artificial. We have deprived nature of its independence, and that is fatal to its meaning. Nature's independence *is* its meaning; without it there is nothing but us" (p. 58).

But if nature has ended, then it isn't clear any longer what environmentalism is supposed to protect. Without nature, an environmental theory or practice oriented toward nature's protection has nothing left to do: the game is up, and we (and nature) have simply lost. If McKibben is right, defending nature makes no more sense than defending the Holy Roman Empire or rooting for the Brooklyn Dodgers. His argument appears deeply pessimistic (and self-defeating) in its implications; it can only lead to sadness about what has been lost, but not to any positive environmental policies at all. After the end of nature, it seems, there's not much for environmental thinking to do except to mourn, and perhaps to think about what was lost and why. For nature once ended cannot be restored.

One possible response to this problem, of course, is to deny that McKibben is right: nature, although threatened, is not quite gone, one might say, and environmental philosophy's role is to protect what's left of it. There are problems with this response—not the least of which is that he probably *is* right—but I won't go into them here. Rather, I would like to consider a different possible response to the pessimism his thesis seems to generate, one that instead of denying nature's end rather wonders why the end of nature should entail the end of environmental concern. Supposing for the sake of argument that his thesis were unquestionably true, would the fact that nature has ended mean that environmental considerations had suddenly become irrelevant—for example, that further global warming ought not to be prevented or that the dumping of toxic wastes into waterways is now fine? Wouldn't one expect a good environmentalist to continue to oppose those processes—and not only for anthropocentric reasons but because of what they do *to the environment,* "unnatural" though that environment would now turn out to be? If the entire environment has become a built one, wouldn't we then need to develop an *environmentalism of the built environment?* Indeed, one might even start to wonder whether the emphasis on the protection of *nature* could actually be an obstacle, nowadays, to clear environmental thinking. If most or all of the world that "environs" us is *not* natural, then shouldn't it be the built environment, and not nature, that is the focus of our environmental concern? Mightn't worry about nature seem more like a diversion from the central issues? Such considerations, perhaps surprisingly, suggest that environmental thought need not be oriented toward the protection of nature and that instead there might be a role for *environmental philosophy after the end of nature.*

Of course, at this point a key question—which is the question underlying the issues discussed in this volume—will obviously be what is meant by *nature?* When McKibben says that nature has ended, it's clear what he has in mind: *nature* means the world independent of human beings and human action. The "natural" temperature of a location, for example, is the temperature it would be if no human beings had affected it; conversely, if its temperature is the consequence of humans burning fossil fuels, then it is not natural. Yet there is an obvious problem with defining the natural as that which is other than the human: for aren't humans themselves natural? There's something oddly pre-Darwinian about the idea that human action removes objects from nature and makes them unnatural. The human species and its behaviors presumably evolved through the same sorts of biological processes as other species. If this is so, it is unclear why the consequences of those behaviors deserve to be called "unnatural." If humans are natural, then their burning fossil fuels would seem to be natural too, hard to distinguish in terms of naturalness (though doubtless more consequential for the environment) from the activities other animals or plants or microbes engage in. The dams of beavers and the webs of spiders are presumably natural; why are the dams built by humans or the polyester fabrics woven by them not so? Indeed, don't many environmental thinkers insist that humans are *part* of nature and claim as well that it is our *failure* to see ourselves as part of it that leads to the hubris and arrogance whose ultimate consequence is environmental disaster?

One way to answer this (pretty standard and pretty obvious) objection is to point out, as John Stuart Mill already did, that the word *nature* has at least two distinct meanings and that the objection here depends on conflating them (1963, pp. 373–75). On the one hand, we commonly use the word *nature* to mean simply the totality of the physical world subject to the ordinary forces described by physics and chemistry and evolutionary biology, and in this sense human beings, like every other species, are surely natural. The contrast term to "natural" in this sense would be "supernatural," meaning something that somehow exceeds or escapes the world of ordinary physical processes. (And the extension of the term might well be empty.) On the other hand, we surely also use the word *nature* in such a way that the contrast term is not *supernatural* but rather *artificial*. A person with a taste for natural foods or a preference for natural fibers, after all, is not someone who prefers her meals or clothing not to have a supernatural origin, but rather someone who prefers them not to involve acts of human making. Thus *nature* in this second sense means exactly what McKibben suggests: the world other than the human one. The first sense of the term is being used when environmental thinkers worry that humans have forgotten that they are part of nature, but it is the second sense that McKibben is using when he worries that nature has ended. The term is simply ambiguous, and what looks like a contradiction is really the result of the ambiguity.

Clarifying the ambiguity, however, does not fully solve the difficulties. If environmental theory is supposed to tell us something normative about our relationship to nature, it isn't clear that *either* of these meanings of the word will be very helpful. For, as Mill pointed out, in the first sense (where nature is everything in the physical world), *everything* we do and make is natural; in the second (where nature is the non-human), *nothing* is. In neither case can we make much sense out of claims, for instance, that certain human practices or products are more "natural" than others: we either are already guaranteed to be fully natural or else we are guaranteed, by definition, to be nature's opposite. In neither case can we do anything to change this situation.

Protecting nature seems problematic in each case as well. If nature means the nonhuman world, then humans could protect it only by abstaining from having anything to do with it, perhaps by enforcing the boundary between "natural" and "built" environments as stringently as possible. This is an odd conclusion, first of all because if McKibben is right, then it's already too late—the boundary has been breached, nature is gone—but secondly because even if he isn't, such a position seems to have nothing to say about what happens on *this* side of the boundary (where we actually live), leaving us curiously free to engage in any environmental depredations we wish to undertake. If, by contrast, nature simply means (as Mill puts it) "the sum total of all phenomena," then working to protect it seems point-less, because in fact nothing humans do could harm it (1963, p. 374). Nuclear power plants and toxic waste dumps are no less natural than beaver dams or spider webs; the atmospheric consequences of global warming and chlorofluoro-carbon use are no less natural than those of photosynthesis or respiration. If na-ture simply means the physical world, then nature is really in no danger—although *we* might be, and so might some of the other entities found within that world. (But note that a list of "natural" entities so endangered would have to include not only animals and plants but also, for example, buildings and appliances.)

Still, pointing out that *nature* has two meanings, and can refer either to every-thing in the world or to everything in the world other than human beings, does seem to rescue McKibben's argument from the objection that it forgets that hu-man beings are natural too. Let's use the capitalized *Nature* to refer to the first, broader sense of the word, and lower-case *nature* to refer to the second, narrower one. Humans then are doubtless part of Nature, we could say, but still are capable of ending nature. Yet to put it this way is to notice a doubt arising: is McKibben *really* more worried about nature than he is about Nature? More generally, is the goal of environmentalism the protection of nature or is it rather the protection of Nature? And which, by the way, is to be identified with the *environment,* the world environing us? Drawing the distinction between the two meanings solves an apparent difficulty with environmental theory's repeated invocation of "na-ture," but it isn't clear that this leaves environmental theory in a better situation.

For notice that if it is nature in the narrow sense that we are concerned with, then calling certain human actions "unnatural" will no longer depend on discov-ering that they harm Nature but rather will simply be a matter of definition. Hu-man actions will be unnatural not because of what they do to the world but merely because they are actions performed by humans. The word "nature" is here simply stipulatively defined as excluding the human; we can no longer be criticized for acting unnaturally, because the claim that any particular human action is un-natural turns out to be analytic. The strong distinction between nature and the human world and the claim that the latter world is unnatural turn out to be valid by definition, *not* because of the discovery that there are empirically significant differences between the nonhuman world and the human one or because the former world is somehow more genuinely Natural than the latter. When McKib-ben writes that "nature's independence *is* its meaning," he certainly seems to be talking about (lower-case) nature, but when he laments the *end* of nature, it isn't always clear what he has in mind. He writes, for instance, that one of the dismaying consequences of the end of nature is that "we can no longer imagine that we are part of something larger than ourselves" (1989, p. 83). But if nature's independence is its meaning—if it is non-human nature and not Nature as a whole that he is worried about—then in what sense could we ever have imagined that we were *part* of it?

When nature is defined as that which is separate from human beings, the claim that human action destroys nature turns out to be an analytic truth. But analytic truths scarcely seem like good candidates on which to found an ethical or political critique; they are not usually things we bemoan or condemn. Nor, of course, are they things that become true, or more true, over time: it makes little sense, for instance, to say that capitalism or technology or anthropocentric arrogance or modernism have made them true. Yet isn't that what much critical environmental thinking wants to argue? Those who criticize the contemporary world for what it has done, or is doing, or threatens to do, *to* nature, it seems to me, do not intend to be expressing analytic truths. They believe, correctly I think, that the effects of human activity on the world over the past century or two have been baleful and destructive, and they believe that different sorts of human activity might produce effects that are less baleful and destructive. But then it cannot be *nature* in the lower-case sense that they think is being destroyed.

One could, after all, stipulatively define a different term to refer to the complementary concept of *any* species—*shmature*, perhaps, to refer to the world independent of the actions of shrimp or *bature* to the world independent of the actions of beavers. Then it would surely be true that wherever shrimp swam or wherever beavers built dams shmature or bature would be destroyed. Yet to make such definitions would be silly, and to lament the destruction thereby defined into existence would be even sillier. Of course a world that shrimp or beaver had *taken over*, spreading and overpopulating like kudzu, would likely be ecologically disastrous. But note that the problem then would be the harm to Nature, to the world that we *share* with beavers and shrimp, not to shmature or bature. Isn't *that* what environmentalists worry about when they worry about the effect of human action on the world—the end of Nature, not of nature? And in warning us about it, aren't they concerned about a kind of destruction that the right sort of environmental policies have a chance to prevent or to repair—not one that occurs inevitably, no matter which policies we pursue, as a matter of *definition*?

To be unhappy about the replacement of nature by a humanized world, I am suggesting, one must be able to point to some (presumably lamentable) empirical characteristic that the natural world possesses that a humanized one does not.

But then that characteristic cannot without begging the question be its natural-ness *alone,* if naturalness simply means nonhumanness. Thus it cannot justifiably be just the end of (lower-case) *nature* that bothers McKibben: there must be some-thing that the humanization of nature actually *harms,* and it is that something—is it capitalized Nature?—that he is really concerned to protect. That human beings can (but need not) destroy nature, that they can (but often do not) live in accor-dance with nature, that nature could (but often does not) serve as a normative model for their actions—these are all meaningful ideas, and yet if "nature" is being defined in the stipulative sense as that which is simply other than human action, then none of these ideas make much sense at all because they all either affirm or deny (pointlessly, in either case) what the definition of nature analyti-cally guarantees to be true.

If nature means the nonhuman, then the "end of nature" through human ac-tion can neither be criticized nor prevented, because its occurrence is a matter of definition, not of choice. And so, it seems to me, an environmental theory that wants to protect nature cannot intend by *nature* that second, lower-case, mean-ing. The assertion that "human action is ending nature" must be a synthetic one, which is to say there must be some *matter of fact* about human beings that re-moves their actions and the results of those actions from nature, for reasons that are more than definitional. So "nature" in the last sentence cannot mean nature in the lower-case sense. But it cannot easily mean Nature in the capitalized sense either because in that sense humans are supposed to be *part* of Nature as "the sum total of all phenomena", and it is hard to see how they could end *that.*

Now *nature* has at least one other common signification—surely relevant here—whereby it refers neither to the sum of all phenomena nor to the specifically nonhuman world but rather to the world of *life.* We speak of someone deciding to leave the city and move into the country as a person who wants to be closer to nature, and here we clearly do not mean by *nature* either the physical world as a whole (because otherwise she'd already be there, in the city) or the nonhuman world (because otherwise she'd never get there, no matter how far she moved). *Nature* in this sense means the *biological* world, the world of flora and fauna, the biosphere. There's not much nature in the city, we say, with the exception of parks or weeds growing between cracks in the sidewalk.

But this third meaning of *nature* surely doesn't solve the problem, for humans are of course alive too and so are still fully natural even in this sense. Is it possible, though, that the definition of "nature" we have in mind is one in which living human beings themselves are natural but their *products* are not? The contrast term to *natural* in Mill's second sense, remember, was *artificial,* not *human.* The end of nature in this sense would mean not the transformation of nature into something human so much as its transformation into something *made* by humans—an artifact.

To say that humans are natural but the products they create are not (are artificial) sounds plausible, but a little thought suggests that there is something odd about it. For one thing, among the products humans create are other humans—and I'm not talking about cloning or IVF or similar examples, I'm talking about ordinary sexual reproduction. A baby conceived in the traditional way *is* after all a human product, and this fact suggests that not all human products, nor all human actions, are unnatural. When we exhale, when we defecate, when we make babies, the objects we produce are not typically called artificial or unnatural. It thus seems as though *some* of the behaviors through which humans produce new objects in the world are natural while others are not. We emit carbon dioxide into the atmosphere when we exhale, and we also emit it when we build and drive automobiles powered by fossil fuels. Why is the one sort of emission called natural while the other is artificial and said to threaten the end of nature? The carbon dioxide produced by human respiration surely has some (albeit small) effect on the overall heat absorption of the atmosphere; global temperatures are different from what they would be if no humans were around to breathe. Yet those effects are considered to be natural ones, not different from the effects on global temperatures of the respiration of other animals, or of plant photosynthesis. What distinguishes, then, our natural products from those that are artificial?

Is the distinction one between biological and nonbiological products? If by this is meant that our natural products are those that are themselves alive, the examples of defecation and respiration are sufficient to refute the idea. Is the distinction rather between those products made of organic materials and those that are not? But plastics are made of such materials, as are most "artificial" flavorings and colorings. Or is it the biological character of the *processes* involved that distinguishes natural human products from artificial ones? But much will now depend on what "biological" means. Why is respiration a biological process and not the collection and combustion of fossil fuels? The danger of circularity here is strong: why can't technological methods be understood as biological ones? To say they can't requires having decided ahead of time that technology isn't natural, which begs the very question in dispute. (And note of course that exhalation can be technologically mediated too—most obviously in the case of people who need mechanical assistance with breathing, but in other cases as well. If the quantity of carbon dioxide I exhale increases because I am running on a treadmill, does the additional carbon dioxide now count as an artificial greenhouse gas?) In the course of biological evolution, various organisms have developed various strategies to get around in the world. The processes by which spiders build webs and beavers build dams are surely biological—why not the processes by which humans build automobiles?

Rather than drawing the distinction between natural and unnatural human actions by appealing to biology, one might try appealing instead to the role played by *intention* in the action. We can choose whether to engage in technologically mediated actions like driving cars; respiration or defecation, on the other hand, seem not to be matters of choice, and that might be a reason for calling the latter actions "natural" ones. But many children are born because their parents specifically intended to make them, and we would not want to call artificial someone whose conception was consciously planned by his or her parents. A woman may choose to become pregnant and bear a child, just as she may choose to burn fossil fuels to drive a car. If the role of human intention in producing an object determines whether that object is natural or not, then it is hard to see why the baby she bears is any less artificial than the carbon dioxide her automobile emits. It is true that sometimes the pregnancy does not come to pass despite the actions the hopeful parents engage in to cause it, but sometimes one's car will not run either, despite one's best attempts to start it. Similarly, although it is true that once the pregnancy begins, processes are set into motion that the mother cannot fully control (but which her intentional actions may still affect), it's also the case that once one starts one's car and gets it moving, processes are set in motion that are not fully controllable either (but again which one's intentional actions may surely influence).

Even defecation, an act of nature par excellence, is not in truth so entirely lacking in intentionality. Toilet training, for example, is the process of educating a child in choosing where and when to engage in it. It's true I have no choice whether to defecate or not, but when and where I do so is typically up to me. The truth is that all these actions—becoming pregnant, driving an automobile, even defecating—involve a complicated mixture of intentional and unintentional elements. The trouble with identifying the distinction between natural and artificial human behaviors with the distinction between unintentional and intentional ones is that it fails to acknowledge this complexity and instead treats intentional actions as though they took place somewhere outside the ordinary world of Nature. But the capacity to act intentionally in fact is part of that world; it is a capacity that has evolved in human beings in accordance with standard Darwinian processes, just as the capacity to fly has evolved in birds. Why should the exercise of the former capacity remove an act or its product from nature, while the exercise of the latter does not? Humans act intentionally *in* Nature, not outside of it.

The appeal to intention here, however, should be the tip-off as to what is really going on in these (repeatedly unsuccessful) attempts to distinguish "natural" human products from "artificial" ones. The (familiar) territory we have entered is the territory of Cartesianism. The dualism being posited between humans and nature derives from a dualism within human beings themselves. Humans, it turns out, are inwardly divided; they have two sides, a "natural" side that connects them with the rest of the world of nature and another side, associated with thought and intention, that separates them from it. The distinction between natural and artificial human products is really the distinction between those products we produce using our minds and those we produce using (merely) our bodies. It is the human body that is natural, and so too are that body's products: babies, exhalations, feces. But the mind is something other than the body; its products are different and somehow stand outside the world of nature. When *thought* is employed in the production of something, the product is thereby rendered "artificial" and not natural.

The familiar dualism at work here is one that has been pretty thoroughly discredited and that few philosophers explicitly hold today. It is also pre-Darwinian; rather than seeing thought or intention as themselves capacities that have *evolved* naturally, it treats them as ontologically distinct, as if they had arisen independently of the processes that have led to the capacities of all the other species in the world. Yet despite its philosophical and biological deficiencies, such a dualism does seem to underlie the conception of nature as distinct from the artificial that McKibben (and many others) take for granted. Such a conception, it turns out, functions less as an account of what *nature* is than as an account of what human beings are: creatures who transcend nature, and transcend it because of their minds.

But then those, like McKibben, who employ that conception of nature are not using the word in any way different from those who use it to mean what I have called Nature. For them the two meanings of the word I suggested—Nature as everything in the world and *nature* as everything other than the human—collapse into one: *nature* does mean everything in the (physical) world, but now it turns out that humans live, in part anyhow, in another world. So when McKibben and others say that human beings might end nature, it is indeed Nature that they must mean. I said earlier that the contrast term to *natural* could be either *supernatural* or *artificial,* depending on which sense was being employed, but now the two latter terms turn out to be connected: the reason that (some) human products are called artificial is that human beings *are* (in part) supernatural. Human activity, or at least that kind of human activity in which we employ our minds (and not just our reproductive organs or our digestive systems), is somehow outside of Nature, outside of the ordinary physical world. So the claim that human action harms nature, that human action could conceivably end nature (or already has), is indeed a claim about Nature in the sense of the "sum of all (physical) phenomena"—a sum from which mental or intentional action has been *excluded*—and not the sort of definitional claim about nature discussed earlier.

More specifically, it is a metaphysical claim. If the harm to nature that humans did were any sort of empirical harm, anything that scientific investigation could uncover, then for just that reason the harm would itself be *part of* Nature and so would in fact be no harm *to* Nature at all, though doubtless perhaps a harm to particular entities *within* Nature. Thus, for instance, when it is suggested that human action is unnatural because it violates the finely tuned balance that characterizes nature, the suggestion only makes sense if nature is indeed characterized by such balance: but if human action violates that balance, then apparently nature is not so characterized, unless we have decided beforehand and for other reasons that the effects of human action on nature are not themselves natural. (It would be like saying that birds are unnatural because nature—with the exception of birds, of course—is marked by flightlessness.) Or if it is asserted that the transformative impact of humans on nature is on a scale so radically different from that of other species as to render it unnatural, again this makes sense only if the global impact of natural species can be shown always to remain within certain limits—but of course it cannot be shown to do this unless we have decided antecedently that the impact of human actions is not to be counted in the determination of what the limits are. The argument here is perfectly general; we can't decide whether humans are natural or not by observing nature, because before observing we would need to decide whether humans themselves are part of what is to be observed. But if the dualist claim that humans are at least in part unnatural cannot be a matter of empirical observation, then (if it is not merely a matter of definition) it must be a matter of a metaphysical assumption. It is not a *discovery* about the human impact on nature, but rather a metaphysical presupposition about it.

When environmental thinkers distinguish nature from the human, I am suggesting, this is not because it is possible to discover in the world some ontologically significant difference between those things humans have transformed and those that they have not. Rather, this view begins by *assuming* the existence of such a difference—begins, that is, by assuming that humans are distinct from nature, typically because of their mental capacities—and then uses that assumption to *justify* the claim that that which humans have made or done (the *artificial*) can be ontologically distinguished from the *natural*. The position does not (although it often claims to) posit a species-neutral criterion of naturalness and then notice with regret that the actions and products of one particular species (our own) fail to satisfy it. Rather, it starts by assuming that humans are (partly) unnatural and then looks for a criterion that confirms the assumption. Far from being a discovery about nature, I would argue, the claim that certain acts and products are unnatural is in fact the expression of a certain a priori metaphysical view about human beings. The dualism here is presupposed, not argued for.

And it is hard to avoid the conclusion that this dualism is also fundamentally anthropocentric. Humans stand in an absolutely unique and distinctive relation to nature, according to this view: alone of all the species in the world, their acts have the special ability to move something out of the natural realm entirely, because they possess qualities of reason that themselves transcend nature. This surely is an impressive and metaphysically unique species, one set off ontologically from every other. Why should this sort of view not be called anthropocentric? It is true that this is an anthropocentrism with the signs reversed, in which humans turn out to be unique in that they are uniquely dangerous, capable of visiting a kind of ontological harm on nature of which no other species is capable. The human mind no longer looks here like the crown of creation but rather like a dangerous exotic whose appearance poses a metaphysical peril to nature and its independence. Yet underneath the surface misanthropy, this view of humans remains remarkably similar to that found in traditional triumphalist anthropocentrism: here, too, we humans are viewed as metaphysically distinctive, possessing (because of our reason) extraordinary characteristics that render us singular among all living creatures. The human mind, seemingly *not* a product of ordinary evolutionary processes (because how otherwise could it allow us to "transcend" nature?), appears to this dualism as something sui generis. Aldo Leopold described the land ethic as calling on humans to see ourselves as a "plain member" of the land community, not as its "conqueror," but isn't it exactly as a conqueror, albeit a dangerous conqueror who must be resisted, that human beings appear on this account?

The distinction between humans and nature that seems crucial to much environmental thinking, I am suggesting, depends on a philosophically and biologically untenable dualism that treats human beings as exceptional creatures that somehow transcend the natural. And notice that the problems here are not solved by asserting that the human/nature dualism is not to be understood as absolute but rather involve a continuum, or admit of degrees. It's surely true that when employing the sense of nature as "independent of the human," we tend to speak of degrees of naturalness. But although this fact is sometimes mentioned as if it showed that the dualism posited by such a view of nature does not perniciously remove human beings from the natural order, it shows no such thing. Recasting a binary opposition as a continuum doesn't render it less dualistic, it only extends the dualism along an axis whose poles (even if reached only asymptotically) remain fundamentally opposed to each other. Why is *naturalness* measured along an axis whose negative pole is the human? Human beings here are still anthropocentrically picked out as animals with the remarkable ability to remove items from nature. The fact that this removal is always partial and takes place by degrees does not transform the fundamentally dualist (and anthropocentric) character of the position.

I have been indicating some of the reasons why it is essential to develop a "post-naturalist" environmental philosophy—an environmental philosophy after the end of nature. This is not only because McKibben might be right—nature might already have ended—and yet there remains a lot for environmental philosophers to do. Nor is it only because the end of nature might be something that has always already happened and therefore might be something we need to learn how to think about without nostalgia. Both these reasons at least assume we know what nature is, and know in particular how and why to distinguish it from the human. What I have argued, however, is that even this may not be so clearly true. Not only might nature the thing have ended, but the *concept* of "nature" might be such an ambiguous and problematic one, so prone to misunderstanding and so riddled with pitfalls, that its usefulness for a coherent environmental philosophy will turn out to be small indeed. We have seen the difficulties in the concept, especially when it is employed dualistically to mean something like (but not exactly, it turns out) "that which is independent of the human"; it seems to require continual modification, it frequently issues in antinomies, it produces a series of paradoxes, and most of all its employment seems to commit one to an essentially Cartesian anthropocentrism that fits uncomfortably with the other theoretical commitments most environmental philosophers typically defend. If we find ourselves unable even to define what we mean by the term *nature,* and if our attempts to define it involve us in metaphysical thickets that philosophers over the past two centuries have found it much more reasonable to avoid, then it might be worthwhile to consider whether environmental philosophy would be better off if it dropped the concept altogether.

REFERENCES

McKibben, B. 1989. *The End of Nature.* New York: Anchor.
Mill, J. S. 1963. "Nature." In *Collected Works,* vol. 10. Toronto: University of Toronto Press.

CHAPTER SEVEN

The Appeal to Nature

Bonnie Steinbock, Ph.D.

The appeal to nature as a reason for moral commendation and even moral obligation has existed throughout the ages, beginning with the Stoics and the Epicure-
ans. It appears in Roman law, canon law, and in modern times in international
law. In "On Nature," John Stuart Mill observes, "That any mode of thinking, feeling, or acting, is 'according to nature' is usually accepted as a strong argument for
its goodness . . . and the word unnatural has not ceased to be one of the most vi-
tuperative epithets in the language" (1904, p. 47).

But is there any justification for an appeal to nature or what is natural? Mill's
analysis is startlingly contemporary. His view that "conformity to nature, has no
connection whatever with right and wrong" (p. 68) has been adopted and refor-
mulated by contemporary philosophers, including Allen Buchanan (2009), David
DeGrazia (2005), Ronald Green (2007), and John Harris (1998). On the other side
of the issue are several other contemporary philosophers, including Leon Kass,
who until recently chaired the President's Council for Bioethics (2002), Francis
Fukuyama (2002), Jürgen Habermas (2003), Erik Parens (1995), and Michael Sandel (2007). In this chapter, I examine the arguments put forth by opponents and
supporters of the appeal to nature or the natural. I conclude that such appeals can
have a role in moral reasoning, but not the robust role often claimed for it. While
nature does and should have value for us, nature is not the source of substantive
moral rules. It is, rather, subject to moral assessment.

Let us begin with Mill's arguments for the absolute rejection of nature as normative. He distinguishes between two main senses of nature:

1. "Nature means the sum of all phenomena, together with the causes which produce them; including not only all that happens, but all that is capable of happening" (1904, p. 44). When we talk about the laws of nature, we are using nature in this first sense.

2. Nature as opposed to Art, and natural to artificial—whatever takes place without the voluntary agency of man is nature.

Which sense of nature is intended in the assertion that nature should be our guide? Clearly, it cannot be the first sense of the term, because, as Mill writes, "in this signification, there is no need of a recommendation to act according to nature, since it is what nobody can possibly help doing, and equally whether he acts well or ill" (p. 49). Because it is not possible to avoid conforming one's action to the laws of nature, it makes no sense to recommend that one ought to act in accordance with nature.

Of course, we should study the laws of nature (what is likely to occur if we act in certain ways) and use that knowledge as a guide to action. To do otherwise would be foolish indeed. Mill writes, "a person who goes into a powder magazine either not knowing, or carelessly omitting to think of, the explosive force of gunpowder, is likely to do some act which will cause him to be blown to atoms in obedience to the very law which he has disregarded" (p. 51). However, to study nature is not to follow nature or to find in nature behavioral norms.

What about the second sense of Nature, in which the natural is opposed to the artificial? Mill argues that this too provides no guide to action. All of human history is an intervention with the natural order in an attempt to improve our lives. Civilization itself is a triumph of the artificial over the natural. Mill writes, "If the artificial is not better than the natural, to what end are all the arts of life? To dig, to plough, to build, to wear clothes, are direct infringements of the injunction to follow nature" (p. 51). Every human intervention into the course of nature, from the draining of marshes to prevent outbreaks of malaria to the vaccination of children to prevent measles and polio, is unnatural in the sense of being the product of human invention.

Moreover, if we were to imitate what occurs in Nature in our own actions, we would be committing the greatest crimes. As Mill explains, "In sober truth, nearly all of the things which men are hanged or imprisoned for doing to one another, are nature's every day performances . . . Nature impales men, breaks them as if on the wheel, casts them to be devoured by wild beasts, burns them to death, crushes them with stones like the first Christian martyr, starves them with hunger, freezes them with cold, poisons them by the quick or slow venom of her exhalations, and has hundreds of other hideous deaths in reserve, such as the ingenious cruelty of a Nabis or a Domitian never surpassed" (p. 56).[1] Mill concludes, "Either it is right that we should kill because nature kills; torture because nature tortures; ruin and devastate because nature does the like; or we ought not to consider at all what nature does, but what it is good to do" (p. 57).

Why then would anyone think that there is a connection between what is natural and what has moral worth? Mill suggests that this stems from a "vague notion" that nature is "God's work, and as such perfect," that nature is a manifestation of the Creator's will, "a sort of finger-posts pointing out the direction which things in general, and therefore our voluntary actions, are intended to take" (p. 53). Because of this association between the Creator and his creation, people have a tendency "to regard any attempt to exercise power over nature . . . as an impious effort to usurp divine power" (p. 53). Thus, every new interference with the natural order has been viewed with suspicion; "each new one was doubtless made with fear and trembling, until experience had shown that it could be ventured on without drawing down the vengeance of the Gods" (p. 52).

The idea that God will zap you if you mess with his creation is crude, and it surely provides no lesson for us today. However, a related, though a more plausible and more sophisticated view persists, namely, that it is unseemly for humans to presume to remake nature according to their own desires and purposes. This idea is expressed by Michael Sandel in *The Case against Perfection* (2007). Sandel argues that enhancement and genetic engineering "represent a kind of hyper-agency, a Promethean aspiration to remake nature, including human nature, to serve our purposes and satisfy our desires. The problem is not the drift to mechanism but the drive to mastery. And what the drive to mastery misses, and may even destroy, is an appreciation of the gifted character of human powers and achievements" (pp. 26–27).

What precisely does Sandel mean by the idea of giftedness? He writes, "To acknowledge the giftedness of life is to recognize that our talents and powers are not wholly our own doing, not even fully ours, despite the efforts we expend to develop and to exercise them" (p. 27). This seems clearly true; no one chooses either his genetic inheritance or the environment in which he develops. But what is the moral significance of that? The fact that we are all subject to the genetic and environmental lottery says nothing about what we may do to improve it. Sandel goes on to say, "It is also to recognize that not everything in the world is open to any use we may desire or devise." This too seems unobjectionable, but to say this is just to say that our desires and devices are subject to moral criticism. It gives no reason for thinking that nature is the criterion by which to assess human desires or human projects. Sandel also says that appreciation of the giftedness of life "constrains the Promethean project and conduces to a certain humility" (p. 27). If the humility to which he refers is the recognition of our limited knowledge and the ways in which our interventions can make things worse, Sandel clearly has a point. Human arrogance and shortsightedness have resulted in vast environmental damage, of which global warming is only the most recent manifestation. Still, it is unclear what Sandel means by the "Promethean project" or why he thinks it needs to be constrained. According to legend (as recounted on Wikipedia), Prometheus played a trick on Zeus. He placed two sacrificial offerings before him: ox meat hidden inside an ox's stomach ("something nourishing hidden inside a displeasing exterior"), and the ox's bones wrapped in "glistening fat" ("something inedible hidden inside a pleasing exterior"). Zeus chose the latter, which set a precedent for future sacrifices. From that time onward, humans would keep the meat for themselves and burn the bones wrapped in fat as an offering to the gods. Angered by this second-rate sacrifice, Zeus hid fire from humans in retribution. Prometheus, who seems to have had a soft spot for humans, then stole fire from Zeus and gave it back to humans for their use. As punishment, Zeus had Prometheus chained to a rock where his liver was eaten daily by an eagle. In some versions of the story, Prometheus not only gave humankind fire but also taught them the arts of civilization such as writing, mathematics, agriculture, medicine, and science. If this is the "Promethean project," surely it is not objectionable, nor should it be constrained. Indeed, the hero of the story is Prometheus, the benefactor of humankind, while Zeus comes off as both choleric and petty.

A more sympathetic reading of Sandel just leaves out the reference to Prometheus. However, we still need to understand precisely what he finds objectionable in the drive to remake nature. Surely Sandel does not think that all interventions into nature are bad. It is *hyper*-agency, *overdoing* the intervention into nature that is worrisome. A good reason to approach human interference into the natural order with caution, if not fear and trembling, stems from the recognition of human fallibility, along with all-too-human failings of pride. An example is the resurgence of breast-feeding. In the 1940s, most middle-class women bottle-fed their babies, partly out of prudishness, but also they were encouraged by their doctors in the belief that formula was better for babies than breast milk, precisely because it was not a mere artifact of nature but had been scientifically determined to give infants exactly what they needed in the way of nutrients. Today, this simplistic faith in science seems touchingly naïve, as well as hubristic. As any obstetrician or pediatrician will tell you, human breast milk is better for human infants than cow's milk. But is the correct explanation for this fact that breast milk is "natural"? Certainly, evolution plays a part in the explanation for the superiority of breast milk: If mother's milk were not good for babies, the species probably would have died out. However, we should not overemphasize evolution's ability to create what is best. As Daniel Dennett reminds us, evolution is "a tournament of blind trial and error from which improvements automatically emerge" (Dennett, 2005). While it can generate "breathtakingly ingenious designs," the trial and error process also produces adaptations that are clumsy, pointless, or even counterproductive. The eye is a perfect example: "Brilliant as the design of the eye is, it betrays its origin with a tell-tale flaw: the retina is inside out. The nerve fibers that carry the signals from the eye's rods and cones (which sense light and color) lie on top of them, and have to plunge through a large hole in the retina to get to the brain, creating the blind spot. No intelligent designer would put such a clumsy arrangement in a camcorder, and this is just one of hundreds of accidents frozen in evolutionary history that confirm the mindlessness of the historical process" (Dennett, 2005).

This suggests that we cannot conclude that "breast is best" simply from the fact that it is the product of thousands of years of evolution. At the same time, we know from scientific studies that there are real advantages to breast milk over cow's milk or formula. For example, breast milk contains nutrients, such as long-chain polyunsaturated fatty acids, which are abundant in breast milk but not in cow's milk or most formulas and, it seems, contribute to intellectual development (Mahoney, 2002). Recently, researchers discovered a genetic reason for the higher IQ scores of breast-fed over bottle-fed children: a gene variant found in the vast majority of people (90 percent of the population). Breast-fed children with this gene variant scored an average of seven points higher on IQ tests than children nourished on formula or cow's milk, while children with another, less common variation of the gene did not benefit from breast-feeding at all. The results held regardless of family income or parents' IQ (Carey, 2007). If it is the presence of fatty acids in breast milk that accounts for greater intelligence (or more precisely, better scores on IQ tests) in most people, then formula presumably could be improved to include these fatty acids. However, even that would not necessarily make bottle-feeding just as good as breast-feeding because breast-feeding also facilitates a physical and emotional bond between mother and child that may be difficult to replicate with bottle-feeding, which likely also plays a role in increased intelligence. In addition, breast milk passes some of the mother's immunity to disease to the baby, something no formula can do. This is especially important in developing countries, where infant mortality is high. Formula not only is more expensive than breast milk but also runs the risk of infecting infants if mixed with water that is unsafe. It is all of these features that make it true that "breast is best," not the simple appeal to the natural. If breast-feeding did not promote children's physical, emotional, and intellectual development better than bottle-feeding, breast would not be best. (For the children of women who are HIV-positive, breast is not best.)

A related example concerns natural childbirth. Women used to be knocked out with ether or other drugs during labor. This reduced the pain in labor, but at a cost: drugs given to a woman can adversely affect her baby. The advantage of "natural childbirth" is that it does not introduce extraneous elements that may prove harmful. Moreover, because we do not always know what will prove harmful, sticking with what is "natural" reduces the chance of iatrogenically caused harm. A similar explanation is given for the appeal of organic foods. Chemicals that kill bugs may also prove harmful to human health. So one justification for the appeal to nature, as opposed to human artifice, is the unexpected and harmful side effects of human intervention. There are many examples of this: the killing of wolves and mountain lions resulted in the overpopulation of deer. The introduction of DDT created DDT-resistant insects and caused the formation of fragile eggs, leading to the devastation of certain bird populations. There have been many interventions, intended to make our lives better, that have resulted in the destruction of ecosystems, global warming, and other disasters. A reasonable interpretation of the appeal to nature and the natural (and one that is, I think, consistent with Mill's approach) is as a warning against overconfidence in our ability to improve matters with human intervention. Applied to the possibility of genetic enhancement, it grounds "a counsel of prudence to go slowly and to take seriously the possibility that we may unwittingly do damage to ourselves in the pursuit of betterment" (Buchanan, 2009, pp. 148).

By contrast, appeals to nature are illegitimate when they express what Allen Buchanan refers to as "normative essentialism": the idea that it is possible to derive substantive moral rules from reflection on nature, including human nature. Buchanan maintains that the normative essentialist faces a destructive dilemma. Either the concept of human nature is rich and detailed enough to ground the moral rules it claims are entailed, in which case the concept of human nature it relies on is itself controversial, or it provides a concept of human nature that, while thin enough to apply universally without controversy, cannot provide guidance in interesting cases.

Normative essentialism lies at the heart of the objection to reproductive cloning in the report by the President's Council on Bioethics. The council wanted to give an argument against reproductive cloning, stemming from its being "unnatural" or "contrary to human nature," that would not also apply to all of assisted reproduction, which is also clearly "unnatural." It did this by contrasting IVF, which is sexual reproduction in the sense of combining the genes of the father and mother, with cloning, which is asexual. "With IVF, assisted fertilization of egg by sperm immediately releases a developmental process, linked to the sexual union of the two gametes, that nature has selected over millions of years for the entire mammalian line. But in cloning experiments to produce children, researchers would be transforming a sexual system into an asexual one, a change that requires major and 'unnatural' reprogramming of donor DNA if there is to be any chance of success. They are neither enabling nor restoring a natural process" (2002, p. 104).

The council regards the asexual character of cloning as being in itself an objection to reproductive cloning, quite apart from any safety considerations, because it is not a "natural" process, nor does it enable or restore a natural process. But when the council goes on to justify the significance of the natural, in particular, *why* sexual reproduction has a moral significance that asexual reproduction lacks, it can come up with nothing better than misconceptions about cloning and identity, and dubious empirical claims. "By giving rise to genetically new individuals, sexual reproduction imbues all human beings with a sense of individual identity and of occupying a place in this world that has never belonged to another. Our novel genetic identity symbolizes and foreshadows the unique, never-to-be-repeated character of each human life. At the same time, our emergence from the union of two individuals, themselves conceived and generated as we were, locates us immediately in a network of relation and natural affection" (p. 112).

It is not entirely clear what is meant by the symbolism of novel genetic identity. If the claim is that individuals created by somatic cell nuclear transfer would necessarily lack the sense of individual identity that the rest of us have, this has been refuted many times (Brock, 1997; Harris, 1998; Steinbock, 1997, 2006). The clone, or "monoparental child" (Silver, 2002, p. 1040), will be a separate individual, with his or her own unique physical and psychological characteristics. Both environmental and epigenetic factors ensure that no two human individuals are exactly alike. To think that genetic identity determines personal identity, so that two individuals who share a genome would have the same physiognomy or personality, is to fall victim to the fallacy of genetic determinism. Moreover, it is refuted by the example of monozygotic twins, who have a nearly identical genome but clearly are different people, each with his or her own personal and novel identity.[2]

But perhaps I am being overly literal. Perhaps the council is not claiming that clones would not be unique individuals but rather that their lack of a unique genome might affect their sense of being a unique, never-to-be-repeated individual. While identical twins seem to be able to develop such a sense, in spite of having (nearly) the same DNA, the situation might be different for clones because twins live out their lives at the same time. As alike as twins may be in their tastes and talents, they still have to discover their own tastes and develop their own talents. In doing so, they each create their own self. By contrast, a clone's life begins after the donor of the DNA has already reached adulthood. There before his or her eyes is a life already lived. Might this not induce a sense of something less than total uniqueness? After all, children who greatly resemble a parent are sometimes—to their annoyance—told things like, "You look just like your father!" Their response is often, "No, I'm don't! I look like me." Monoparental children presumably would be subject to greater numbers of such comments and therefore might find it psychologically more difficult to find and create their own unique identity.

This is not a silly worry, but it is worth remembering that the development of "narrative identity" (DeGrazia, 2005) predates the modern understanding of genetics. Indeed, it has been alleged that the Aristotelian view of procreation, which held sway until modern times, made the male the sole creator of the embryo and fetus, with the female as gestator merely providing nutrition for its growth. On this model, the father provides active material—just as would happen if a child were cloned from a somatic cell of the rearing father and gestated by the rearing mother. Presumably, being created by one parent (the father) did not give our ancestor identity crises, so it is not obvious why having only one genetic forebear would make the development of a sense of identity problematic for a cloned child. It seems that identity in the narrative sense has nothing to do with understanding that genes come from both parents. Each individual, whether the result of sexual intercourse, IVF, or (should this become possible) cloning, experiences himself or herself as having a life story that is the basis of narrative identity. Moreover, if a cloned child were to think, "I'm not unique, I'm just a clone of my father," we could correct this misunderstanding about identity through education. We could remind the child that genes are only part of narrative identity. Even clones, who get almost all their genes from one parent (there is some mitochondrial DNA in the enucleated egg), would not be a just a copy or a replica because every individual is a unique product of his or her genome interacting with the environment. Indeed, because a clone will be gestated in a different uterus than the provider of its DNA, and grow up in a different family in a different era, we can expect clones to be less alike than monozygotic twins. This should reassure monoparental children.

Another concern relating to identity has to do with the attempt to choose the traits of offspring by genetic manipulation. As we learn more about the genetic bases of physical and emotional characteristics, the possibility of "designing" children looms. Most people are not too concerned with the idea of preventing serious genetic diseases by such intervention at the embryonic stage, safety considerations aside, but many are disturbed at the idea of choosing character traits. Gregory Kaebnick put the worry this way: "They might feel that they had come to be who they were in a way that gave partial credit to somebody else for coming up with the basic design, and so weren't quite their *own*" (e-mail communication, April 8, 2009).

This concern rests on an intuition that if one's genes and related traits are the result of nature, which is to say chance, then they are one's own in a way that they are not if they are the result of someone else's choice. One imagines the child saying to the parent, "*You* wanted me to be musical (or outgoing or brainy). By choosing those traits for me, you infringed my autonomy." However, it seems to me that this thought is incoherent. It imagines that the child's true nature is the genome that existed at conception, which has been changed by parental interference. But why is this genome, which is the result of the genetic lottery, any more true or authentic than one that is chosen? Why would the me that develops from chance be more authentic, more truly me, than the self that develops from genes that were chosen? Admittedly, if my parents chose my genes, then they would be choosing for me. Many of us would rather make our own choices, rather than have others make them for us. However, no one gets to choose his genome. It's either the result of chance or the result of someone else's choice. It just isn't clear why developing a sense of self or a narrative identity is better facilitated by chance than choice.

Consider a child born to two musical parents. The child likely will inherit musical talent, but whether the child becomes a musician depends on whether the child practices and develops that talent. The child might rebel and refuse to have anything to do with music. Genetic inheritance does not determine who or what one becomes. Exactly the same will be true of a child of nonmusical parents who have genetically manipulated the embryo in the hopes of getting a musical child. Both children will have to decide whether to develop the talents bestowed on them; neither has chosen this advantage. Nor has either child grounds for complaint. Both should be grateful for the opportunity they have been given. Of course, if parents attempted to give their children bad traits, traits not likely to help them flourish or live good lives, that would be grounds for complaint. But the complaint would be the kinds of traits chosen, not the act of choosing them or, to be more accurate, of choosing the genes likely to be associated with certain traits.

Moreover, all parents strive to influence our children's traits. Traditionally, this is accomplished by education and example. Is the attempt to influence their traits genetically dramatically different? We should remember that environmental influences, such as nutrition and childrearing methods, make actual changes in the brain. To think that genetic manipulation is more permanent and less susceptible to change than neuronal manipulation (i.e., education) is to fall victim to the fallacy of genetic determinism.

Another objection to choosing our children's genes stems from a fear that if parents are given a choice, they will all choose the same traits for their children, reducing difference and individuality. In a world where genes are chosen, as opposed to provided by nature, perhaps all children will have blond hair and blue eyes, have a talent for soccer, and find it easy to play a musical instrument. Consider the recent trend for Hollywood actresses to look like each other. This was not the case in the 1940s; Bette Davis could not be mistaken for Katharine Hepburn. Today, plastic surgery increasingly makes it difficult to tell one star from another. If appearance could be determined prenatally, perhaps all girls would look like Jennifer Aniston (or like Jennifer Aniston after all the plastic surgery). While such concerns would not warrant state control, any more than plastic surgery is controlled to make sure that people do not end up with the same nose, it would be sad if prenatal interventions resulted in sameness. Diversity of looks, talents, and temperaments enriches our lives and is a value to be protected. I suspect that the pressures on Hollywood actresses would not incline parents toward creating similar children, if only because then the different ones would have a better chance of getting into Harvard! In addition, we know from history that periods of conformity, such as the 1950s, seem to be followed by periods in which nonconformity is valued.

Another reason why the council favored sexual over asexual reproduction is that sexual union "immediately locates each individual in a network of relation and natural affection." As an empirical claim, this is manifestly not true because some children are conceived from rape, a one-night stand, or other encounters that do not give rise to networks of relation and natural affection. Children are born into such networks when assisted reproduction is used, but the relations and affection have nothing to do with genetic connection. Sperm and egg donors typically do not even know of the existence of the child created from their genetic material. Rather, the "network of relation and natural affection" stems from the intention to become parents and is provided by the rearing parents. There is no reason to think that parents who use assisted reproduction have less affection for their children than genetically related parents. Should cloning be proven safe and effective, it could be a useful technique for individuals who wanted a genetic connection with at least one parent and did not want to introduce a third party into their relationship. A couple could create an embryo genetically related to either the man or the woman and then have the woman gestate the embryo and fetus. When that couple brought the baby home from the hospital, that child would be located in a network of relation and natural affection, just as any child born from assisted reproduction, or any adopted child. Thus, neither of the President's Council's reasons for rejecting cloning—that it would necessarily produce a child who had identity problems or who lacked a network of relations and natural affection—are valid.

Finally, the appeal to nature or the natural can result in attitudes that should be rejected as discriminatory and unjust. As Buchanan points out, "The history of prejudice and persecution is replete with normative essentialist claims: homosexuality is unnatural, marriages between the races are unnatural, social equality for inferior and superior types of humans (Aryans and non-Aryans, Nietzschean 'higher-types' and 'lower-types') is unnatural, demeaning (to the superior), etc. That alone should make one suspicious of normative essentialist claims and prompt an insistence that they be backed up with evidence or argument" (2009, p. 146). In the light of this history, we need more than Kass's "wisdom of repugnance" (1997) to inform our judgments about which "unnatural" institutions and arrangements should be rejected. Nor does Sandel's ethic of giftedness provide moral guidance. Such an ethic could be used (undoubtedly has been used) to oppose, for example, contraception. If children are a gift, then parents should be grateful and happy to accept them at any time. This attitude, while still espoused by the Catholic Church, is one that the majority of people (including Catholic married couples) no longer accept, and for good reason. People's lives go better when they have some control over the number and spacing of their children. Having fewer children has been essential for improving the status of women and combating poverty. Nor is there any evidence that the availability of contraception has adversely affected the parent-child relationship.

Does this mean that the ethic of giftedness has no value, or none except as a warning against hubris and overconfidence? The ideal of giftedness points toward a valuable ideal, namely, the natural environment is not only something in which most people delight but also is something toward which we *should have* an attitude of protectiveness, as opposed to exploitation. David Wiggins discusses this view of nature in a paper in which he talks about a farmer's anger at the disappearance from the countryside of the barn owl, partridge, otter, brown hare, cowslip, and marsh marigold, as the result of the industrialization of agriculture.

It is a lament at the disappearance—for which we as a species are directly or indirectly solely responsible (because we caused it)—of all sort of things human beings have loved or delighted in, and might still in the future love or delight in, with the option to find indefinitely many other such things for whose loss we could scarcely imagine ourselves being compensated. Like hedgerows, wetlands, meadows, and the other things for whose loss or devastation the author and many other people find themselves inconsolable, these form one part of the great framework for a life on earth in which (articulately or not, as the case may be) human beings can find meaning. They form one part of the benign aspect of Nature, where Nature may be understood not as that which is free of all trace of our interventions—in England few things could pass such a test—but as that which has not been entirely instrumentalized by human artifice, and as something to be cherished by the farmer or forester in ways that outrun all considerations of profit. (2000, p. 10)

The value the natural world has is, to be sure, a value for us, but it is not, or not only, commercial value, not even to the farmer and forester who profit from working the land or cutting down trees. A world in which there was great economic prosperity but which was so polluted that human beings could not see the stars or enjoy a sunset or hear birds sing would hardly be a world worth living in. And despite what he has to say about the superiority of the artificial to the nature, Mill apparently agrees with this sentiment. Wiggins quotes him on precisely this point: "Nor is there much satisfaction in contemplating the world with nothing left to the spontaneous activity of Nature; with every rood of land brought into cultivation which is capable of producing food for human beings; every flowering waste or nature pasture ploughed up, all quadrupeds or birds which are not domesticated for man's use exterminated as his rivals for food, every hedgerow or superfluous tree rooted out, and scarcely a place left where a wild shrub or flower could grow without being eradicated in the name of improved agriculture" (Mill, 1848, p. 311).

In this passage, we see the notion of limits to human intervention and cultivation, the idea that more is not always better. In the effort to conquer the wilderness, to tame the forest, humankind has displayed a greediness and insatiability that now threatens our very existence. Wiggins opposes this sort of attitude with the idea of "grateful contentment"—"the propensity to cultivate contentment in such good things as the world furnishes, watchfulness on behalf of those good things, and awareness of human limitations such as our ignorance and our imperfect mastery of the nature and social processes we live in the midst of. At this point in the development of the earth, what could be a more reasonable frame of mind?" (p. 30).

Insofar as the appeal to nature is an appeal to humility, grateful contentment with what the natural world offers, and recognition of our responsibility not to despoil the natural world, it is a legitimate aspect of moral discourse. Humility in the face of unknown risks and limited human knowledge is clearly warranted, especially in light of human destruction of fragile ecosystems. Moreover, another aspect of humility is to be awed by the power and beauty of nature. To reduce nature to its commercial value is crass. Finally, the idea of gratitude for the natural world seems a completely appropriate human attitude. But none of this requires us to accept blindly nature as a guide for our actions or to reject something simply on the ground that it is unnatural in the sense of not existing in nature. That something is natural is not in itself a reason for thinking it is good; that it is unnatural is not a reason for thinking that it is bad. And this is true even though much that exists in nature is in fact beautiful and worthy of appreciation and awe. We need not take the Benthamite view that whatever gives people pleasure is equally valuable. Someone who prefers Disneyland's representation of rock formations to Utah's Monument Valley displays a lack of aesthetic sensibility. (Although this is not limited to the natural world; someone who finds the representation of Venice in Las Vegas more beautiful than the real Venice is also a clod.)

How might grateful contentment with what the natural world offers play out in the field of reproduction? Would an ethic of giftedness support the view that amniocentesis or genetic enhancement of offspring is morally wrong, on the grounds that one ought to be happy with what one gets naturally? I doubt it. Although some people might have this sort of preference, and it is, to my mind, a morally permissible preference, by itself it does not support a moral obligation. To the claim that one ought to be happy with what one gets, and therefore that it is wrong to use prenatal testing, one can reasonably reply, "Why? What is wrong with preferring a healthy, normal child?" To show that amniocentesis is morally problematic, one would have to argue that it harms, or discriminates against people with disabilities, or "sends a message" that their lives are of less value. (For a rejection of the disability critique, see Steinbock, 2000.) Similarly, to show that genetic enhancement of offspring is wrong, one would have to show that it distorts the proper parent-child relationship or is incompatible with the right kind of parental love and acceptance. The limit of "giftedness" as an ethic is that it is undiscriminating about which gifts we should gratefully accept and which ones we can legitimately reject or modify.

The appeal to nature may point to values and ideals that ought to be adopted, but it cannot serve as a substitute for moral argumentation in their support.

NOTES

1. Nabis was the last leader of an independent Sparta, and tyrant from 207 to 192 B.C.E. Described by contemporaries as a bloodthirsty ruler who committed acts of shocking brutality and torture, he was eventually assassinated. Domitian was a first-century Roman emperor of the house of Flavia. Though his reign started out moderate, he soon revealed a cruel nature and, in particular, persecuted Jews and Christians. He was murdered by his enemies in the Senate.

2. It turns out that even identical (or monozygotic) twins do not have identical DNA. Science has long known that identical twins develop differences due to differences in the environment, including position in the womb. In recent years, it has been learned that some of the differences between identical twins are due to epigenetic factors, the chemical markers that attach to genes and affect how they are expressed. Identical twins were still considered genetically identical because epigenetics affects only the expression of a gene, not the sequence of the gene itself. However, a recent study shows that monozygotic twins differ at the genetic level in what are known as copy number variations, in which a gene exists in multiple copies or a set of coding

letters in DNA is missing. It is not known whether these changes occur at the embryonic level or as the twins age or both (O'Connor, 2008). Presumably the person who provided a somatic cell for reproductive cloning would differ from his or her clone in copy number variations, as well as in differences due to environment and epigenetic factors.

REFERENCES

Brock, D. 1997. "Cloning Human Beings: An Assessment of the Ethical Issues Pro and Con." In *Cloning Human Beings: Report and Recommendations of the National Bioethics Advisory Commission.* Rockville, Md.
Buchanan, A. 2009. "Human Nature and Enhancement." *Bioethics* 23 (3): 141–50.
Carey, B. 2007. "Mental Abilities: Gene Found to Play Role in Benefits of Breast Milk." *New York Times,* November 6.
DeGrazia, D. 2005. "Enhancement Technologies and Human Identity." *Journal of Medicine and Philosophy* 30:261–83.
Dennett, D. 2005. "Show Me the Science." *Edge: The Third Culture.* www.edge.org/3rd_culture/dennett05/dennett05_index.html.
Fukuyama, F. 2002. *Our Post-Human Future: Consequences of the Biotechnology Revolution.* New York: Farrar, Straus & Giroux.
Green, R. 2007. *Babies by Design: The Ethics of Genetic Choice.* New Haven, Conn.: Yale University Press.
Habermas, J. 2003. *The Future of Human Nature.* Cambridge, U.K.: Polity.
Harris, J. 1998. *Clones, Genes, and Immortality: Ethics and the Genetic Revolution.* Oxford: Oxford University Press.
Kass, L. 1997. "The Wisdom of Repugnance." *New Republic* 216 (22): 17–26.
Mahoney, D. 2002. "Breast-feeding Linked to Higher Adult IQs—Duration of 7–9 Months." *OB/GYN News,* June 15. http://findarticles.com/p/articles/mi_moCYD/is_12_37/ai_87776272.
Mill, J. S. 1848. *Principles of Political Economy.* Vol. 2. London: John Parke.
———. 1904. "On Nature." In *Nature, The Utility of Religion and Theism* [1874]. London: Watts & Co. for the Rationalist Press.
O'Connor, A. 2008. "REALLY?; The Claim: Identical Twins Have Identical DNA." *New York Times,* March 11.
Parens, E. 1995. "The Goodness of Fragility: On the Prospect of Genetic Technologies Aimed at the Enhancement of the Human Species." *Kennedy Institute of Ethics Journal* 5 (2): 141–53.
President's Council on Bioethics. 2002. *Human Cloning and Human Dignity: The Report of the President's Council on Bioethics.* New York: PublicAffairs.
Sandel, M. 2007. *The Case against Perfection: Ethics in the Age of Genetic Engineering.* Cambridge, Mass.: Belknap Press of Harvard University Press.
Silver, L. 2002. "Public Policy Crafted in Response to Ignorance Is Bad Public Policy." *Hastings Law Journal* 53 (5): 1037–47.
Steinbock, B. 1997. "The NBAC Report on Cloning Human Beings: What It Did—and Did Not—Do." *Jurimetrics* 38:39–46.

———. 2000. "Disability, Prenatal Testing, and Selective Abortion." In *Prenatal Testing and Disability Rights,* ed. E. Parens and A. Asch, pp. 108–23. Washington, D.C.: Georgetown University Press.

———. 2006. "Reproductive Cloning: Another Look." In *Law and Life: Definitions and Decisionmaking,* pp. 87–111. The University of Chicago Legal Forum. Chicago: University of Chicago Law School.

Wiggins, D. 2000. "Nature, Respect for Nature, and the Human Scale of Values." *Proceedings of the Aristotelian Society* 100 (1): 1–32.

CHAPTER EIGHT

Thinking like a Mountain

Nature, Wilderness, and the Virtue of Humility

Paul Lauritzen, M.A., Ph.D.

> Ability to see the cultural value of wilderness boils down, in the last analysis, to a question of intellectual humility.
> —ALDO LEOPOLD, *A SAND COUNTY ALMANAC*

Aldo Leopold begins his famous essay "Thinking like a Mountain" by evoking the haunting call of a wolf. "A deep chesty bawl," he writes, "echoes from rimrock to rimrock, rolls down the mountain, and fades into the far blackness of the night. It is an outburst of wild defiant sorrow, and of contempt for all the adversities of the world." Leopold suggests that the cry of the wolf quickens the pulse of all sentient beings, whether in anticipation of a meal from the gleanings of a hunt or in fear of the blood that may be so spilled. "Yet behind these obvious and immediate hopes and fears there lies a deeper meaning, known only to the mountain itself. Only the mountain has lived long enough to listen objectively to the howl of a wolf."

Talk of "thinking like a mountain" is perhaps overly dramatic, but Leopold has a point in suggesting that experience with wilderness may have something to teach us about intellectual humility. Indeed, I want to suggest that the recognition of the need to cultivate certain virtues, especially humility, may stand behind many of the appeals to "nature" that we find in discussions of medical biotechnology, agricultural biotechnology, and environmentalism. To explore the connection among ideas of "wilderness," "nature," and particular virtues, I want to look briefly at two writers who have wrestled with these connections in compelling ways, Cormac McCarthy and Wendell Berry.[1] There are dangers in appealing to writers whose reflections on wilderness and nature are not conducted within the standard frame of bioethical concerns, but perhaps for that very reason there is wisdom to be found in their writings. Or at least that is what I hope to show. Thus, in the first part of this chapter, I will examine Cormac McCarthy's explorations of wilderness motifs. In the second part, I will turn to consider Wendell Berry's appeals to wilderness and nature.

Cormac McCarthy

Although most of McCarthy's work would be instructive for our purposes, the book on which I will primarily focus is the second volume of his border trilogy, *The Crossing*. *The Crossing* is a complex, sprawling work, but for our purposes, part one of the book, which comprises 127 pages, is the core. Set in 1939 in New Mexico, this section tells the story of sixteen-year-old Billy Parham, who with his father and brother sets out to trap a wolf that has begun to prey on cattle in the range. The story opens with a passage that displays the force of McCarthy's writing, as well as his conviction that there is value in closely observing the "natural" world without seeking to bend it to one's will.

Shortly after the family arrives in the valley they will call home, a very young Billy wakes to the howling of wolves in the hills. He decides to take a look. Here is how McCarthy describes the scene:

> When he passed the barn the horses whimpered softly to him in the cold. The snow creaked under his boots and his breath smoked in the bluish light. An hour later he was crouched in the snow in the dry creekbed where he knew the wolves had been. . . .
>
> They were running on the plain harrying the antelope and the antelope moved like phantoms in the snow and circled and wheeled and the dry powder blew about them in the cold moonlight and their breath smoked palely in the cold as if they burned with some inner fire and the wolves twisted and turned and leapt in a silence such that they seemed of another world entire. . . .
>
> There were seven of them and they passed within twenty feet of where he lay. He could see their almond eyes in the moonlight. He could hear their breath. He could feel the presence of their knowing that was electric in the air. They bunched and nuzzled and licked one another. Then they stopped. They stood

with their ears cocked. Some with one forefoot raised to their chest. They were looking at him. He did not breathe. They did not breathe. They stood. Then they turned and quietly trotted on. (1994, p. 4)

Those unfamiliar with McCarthy's work might come upon this passage and expect a kind of sentimental and romanticized nature story to follow. They would be mistaken, for in this novel, as in all his fiction, McCarthy is unflinching in depicting the violence he sees everywhere in nature, including human nature. Nor is he inclined to be elegiac about the loss of a wilderness untrammeled by humans. For McCarthy, the idea of preserving the natural environment cannot accommodate the violence of the earth's history in which species come and go, both with and without human help. What, then, of human technology?

McCarthy has no illusions about the threat that human technology poses for the earth, but in *The Crossing* McCarthy's vision is not totally apocalyptic. Nor is there any choice here; humans can use it thoughtfully or recklessly, but they will use technology. Indeed, we see this early on as Billy and his father seek to trap the wolf using the longspring traps of a legendary wolf trapper, W. C. Echols, whose years of tracking and studying wolves provided a sort of technical expertise. The narrator's ambivalence about these tools is palpable. On the one hand, Billy's relation to the traps is described almost lovingly: "Crouched in the broken shadow with the sun at his back and holding the trap at eyelevel against the morning sky he looked to be truing some older, some subtler instrument. Astrolabe or sextant. Like a man bent at fixing himself someway in the world. Bent on trying by arc or chord the space between his being and the world that was" (p. 22). Echols is admiringly characterized as "about half wolf hisself" (p. 19). On the other hand, there is an ominous quality to the tools of this trade. Echols's vials of scents for bait have the smell of death about them. "In the jars dark liquids. Dried viscera. Liver, gall, kidneys. The inward parts of the beast who dreams of man and has so dreamt in running dreams a hundred thousand years and more. Dreams of that malignant lesser god come pale and naked and alien to slaughter all his clan and kin and rout them from their house. A god insatiable whom no ceding could appease nor any measure of blood" (p. 17). The anthropomorphism of this passage is uncharacteristic, but the concern about the unconstrained and ceaseless use of technology to trap wolves to the point of extinction is not.[2]

The contrast to such unreflective use of technology, then, is Billy Parham's pursuit of the wolf. Although the initial efforts to catch her are unsuccessful, Billy perseveres and eventually traps the wolf. When he does, he realizes the wisdom of the mysterious and oracular hunter, Don Arnulfo, who has cautioned him about the self-absorption of men who see only the immediate "acts of their own hands" and not the larger world in which they act. In dialogue that recalls the opening scene of the book, Arnulfo explains, "If you want to see the wolf, you have to see it on its own ground. If you catch it, you lose it" (p. 46). Although Billy has planned to kill the wolf and goes so far as to raise the rifle to shoot her, in the end he cannot take her life. Instead, he decides to muzzle and tether the wolf in order to return her to the mountains of Mexico from whence she came. For the next seventy-five pages we witness the destructive and bloody fate of the wolf, who, in being caught, has been lost.

Although Billy will not be able to save the wolf or the pups she carries, he is, nevertheless, steadfast in his efforts. Indeed, it is instructive to attend to Billy's doomed attempt to return the wolf to Mexico and thus avoid her killing. For example, although Billy talks to the wolf and sings to her, it is clear that he does not think of her as his property or his pet. At several points in the narrative, Billy insists that she has been entrusted to his care and that he has no intention of treating her instrumentally (see pp. 60, 70, 90, and 110). Indeed, a recurring theme is that Billy could easily treat the wolf as property and make money from her, which is precisely what almost every other character in the book tries to do. For example, several characters offer to buy the wolf; one expects that Billy will sell her hide or collect the bounty for her. When the wolf is confiscated from Billy in Mexico, she becomes part of a sideshow at a fair, where circus-goers pay to see the "man-eating" wolf. Ultimately, she is set to fighting dogs in an old cock-fighting pit, as men from surrounding towns drink and bet and otherwise find amusement in the spectacle. At every point, Billy fiercely resists this instrumentalization of the wolf. He repeatedly rejects offers of money for her and, in the end, he kills her himself rather than allow her to continue to be mistreated in the fighting pit.

The irony, of course, and the point that emerges most forcefully from part one of *The Crossing* is that Billy himself did not foresee and could not control the consequences of his use of the technology of the traps. At the beginning of part one, Billy has gone out without traps, without a rifle, without even his horse, to find and merely watch the wolves. At the end, Billy can only imagine wolves running the range because during the ten years that Billy's family has lived in New Mexico humans have essentially eradicated the wolf. Even the wolf that Billy desperately tried to save has been killed. The closing paragraph of part one is thus a striking contrast to its opening paragraphs: "He squatted over the wolf and touched her fur. He touched the cold and perfect teeth. The eye turned to the fire gave no light and he closed it with his thumb and sat by her and put his hand upon her bloodied forehead and closed his own eyes that he could see her running the mountains, running in the starlight where the grass was wet and the sun's coming as yet had not undone the rich matrix of creatures passed in the night before her . . . He took up her stiff head out of the leaves and held it or he reached to hold what cannot be held, what already ran among the mountains at once terrible and of great beauty, like flowers that feed on flesh" (p. 127).

Let me now quickly shift gears to suggest how reflecting on *The Crossing* may be helpful to our deliberations on appeals to nature in bioethics. I will take as my point of departure a claim that Greg Kaebnick makes in an essay entitled, "Putting Views about Nature into Context: The Case of Agricultural Biotechnology." According to Kaebnick, appeals to "nature" appear to be quite different depending on whether they are made in debates about medical biotechnology, agricultural biotechnology, or environmentalism. "The result," he says, "is that the three domains look to be distinct from each other, and the associated views of nature have little to do with each other" (2007, p. 6). Nevertheless, Kaebnick believes that there may be a commonality among these appeals to nature that is captured by the conviction that there is value in "resisting the urge to re-engineer natural states of affairs."

I take this suggestion to be that although "nature" may be defined in very different ways in each of these domains, and so resist any articulation of a positive definition of the term, we can still ask: What worry stands behind the effort to differentiate the "natural" from the "unnatural"? We can usefully ask a variation of that question in relation to *The Crossing*. Why is such a sharp contrast drawn between the situation of the wolves in New Mexico at the beginning of the narrative compared to that at the end of part one? What should we make of the contrast that is highlighted repeatedly between Billy's attitude to the wolf and the attitude of others in the story?

The answer to these questions is suggested by Leopold's observation that the cultural value of wilderness is that experience with wilderness may help us to cultivate humility. In this regard, perhaps the key figure in part one of the book is the trapper Don Arnulfo. Billy has gone to Arnulfo to get more bait with which to trap the wolf because Arnulfo is thought to know almost as much about catching wolves as Echols. But Arnulfo tells Billy that he cannot help him and that the idea that Echols "knows what the wolf knows before the wolf knows it" is mistaken. The wolf, he says, is unknowable. You can trap a wolf, but then you do not have a wolf; you have only "teeth and fur." Indeed, Arnulfo appears to regard

Billy's quest to trap the wolf as pure folly. It is the folly of assuming that we can impose order on the world short of the grave. Arnulfo is emphatic: "He said that the wolf is a being of great order and that it knows what men do not: that there is no order in the world save that which death has put there. Finally he said that if men drink the blood of God yet they do not understand the seriousness of what they do. He said that men wish to be serious but they do not understand how to be so. Between their acts and their ceremonies lies the world and in this world the storms blow and the trees twist in the wind and all the animals that God has made go to and fro yet this world men do not see. They see the act of their own hand or they see that which they name and call out to one another but the world between is invisible to them" (p. 46).

When we ask how a conception of "nature" or "wilderness" may provide guidance in thinking about environmental issues, the answer that seems to come from *The Crossing* is that attending to this "invisible" world that is obscured in the human quest for mastery may provide us with lessons in humility.[3] In one sense, what emerges from *The Crossing* is thus a view akin to that articulated by Michael Sandel in relation to medical biotechnology. In *The Case against Perfection,* Sandel contrasts the "drive to mastery" with a recognition that human life is a gift to be cherished rather than improved on. The sense in which the moral vision of *The Crossing* is like Sandel's is that it laments the obsessive willfulness, the "hyperagency," as Sandel puts it, that seeks to control everything. There is, says Sandel, "something appealing, even intoxicating about a vision of human freedom unfettered by the given," but that vision of freedom is deeply flawed. It leaves us "with nothing to affirm or behold outside our own will" (2007, pp. 99–100). Indeed, even Billy Parham can be accused of a kind of hubris in thinking that he can trap the wolf and trail it to Mexico with impunity.

Yet it seems to me that McCarthy would be much less sanguine than Sandel about appealing to the givenness of nature as a moral guide. In that respect, the contrasts between "nature" and "culture," "man" and "nature," or "wilderness" and "nonwilderness" are like many of the borders that are transgressed throughout the book. They are shifting boundaries that are dangerous liminal states. Billy notes at one point that the wolf recognizes no border between the United States and Mexico, but of course it is the crossing of this border that leads to the wolf's death. Indeed, the only fixed boundary is death.

If we return to the questions with which we began this section, we can perhaps now state more directly the concern that haunts most of McCarthy's reflections on the natural world and humanity's relationship to it. Recall that the first question concerned the sharp contrast between the range where there is scarcely any boundary between wolves and humans and one where that boundary is sharply enforced. If we in fact attend to the various boundaries that are described throughout the novel, we observe McCarthy's insistence that borders and boundaries are fluid. They are drawn and redrawn, crossed and recrossed. At first, this might suggest that McCarthy will be of little help to our project, for appeals to nature are frequently made in an effort to set limits—to set boundaries—on what humans may legitimately do to the environment or livestock or themselves. Yet McCarthy's vision appears to question the usefulness of such a mindset. We can describe human nature in a way that attempts to draw a boundary that should not be transgressed, but doing so is a bit like trapping a wolf. A wolf in a trap is not a wolf; a human locked into some essential and unchanging nature is not human. At the same time, McCarthy paints an exquisite picture of the fragility of both the natural world and our relationship to this world and to each other. Nowhere is this more beautifully or hauntingly captured than in McCarthy's novel *The Road*.

The Road tells the story of a father and son who have survived what is presumably a nuclear attack on the United States. They wander in a desolate landscape in which "the frailty of everything [was] revealed at last" (2006, p. 24). Uncharacteristically, the book ends on an optimistic note. When the father dies, the son encounters a family that invites the boy to join them. It is one of the few gestures of "humanity" displayed in the book. Despite this optimism, the book ends with a cautionary paragraph that could be said to sum up McCarthy's worldview entire, as one of his characters might say. It is the last paragraph of the book: "Once there were brook trout in the streams in the mountains. You could see them standing in the amber current where the white edges of their fins wimpled softly in the flow. They smelled of moss in your hand. Polished and muscular and torsional. On their back were vermiculate patterns that were maps of the world in its becoming. Maps and mazes. Of a thing which could not be put back. Not be made right again. In the deep glens where they lived all things were older than man and they hummed of mystery" (p. 241).

This is the central worry of *The Crossing*: human overreaching has the potential irrevocably to change the world in ways that humans cannot, or at least do not, begin to comprehend. And some things, when they are changed, cannot be made right again. In exercising our power, whether in relation to the environment or in relation to agricultural or biomedical technology, the appropriate attitudes are awe and respect for the mystery of the world around us. The appropriate virtue is humility. Instead, we act like "a god insatiable whom no ceding could appease."

Wendell Berry

The second writer to whom I turn for help in thinking about appeals to "nature" and "wilderness," Wendell Berry, is a novelist and poet, and, like Cormac Mc-Carthy, he has an impressive list of literary awards. Berry's fiction demonstrates a keen appreciation of the value of nature and wilderness as a school of virtue for his characters, but it is in his remarkable collection of essays that Berry most fully articulates an account of the relationship between nature—significantly not in scare quotes—and virtue.

To appreciate Berry's body of work, one must place it in the context of his life-long commitment to a Jeffersonian agrarian ideal, for much of his writing is occasioned by concern for the decline of rural America and the family farm. Indeed, his ruminations about nature and wilderness are framed in terms of the cultural costs of losing a sense of connection between our bodies and the land they inhabit. We have come to act as if we are not embodied beings with an inextricable connection to the land. We see this in the idea that we have moved to an information economy. But as Berry caustically observes, "the idea that we have now progressed from a land-based economy to an economy based on information is a fantasy" (2005, p. 114). And it is, Berry says, a fantasy that could be fatal. We have so deluded ourselves about our necessary relation to and dependence on the land that we imperil our long-term survival.

Although the cultural critique that Berry offers is spread out over at least a half-dozen volumes, spanning thirty-five plus years, I want to focus primarily on a handful of essays that delineate almost all the major themes in his work.[4] Most of Berry's writing is rooted in his life as a farmer in rural Kentucky, and all of his best work is directly connected to his attempt to understand (and reverse) what he takes to be the dramatic decline in the agrarian ideal in American life. Let us start with his diagnosis of the ills that confront the family farmer in the United States and of how we got in such a condition.

According to Berry, American agriculture has been in decline at least since the end of World War II. He recognizes that the idea that American agriculture is in decline will likely appear counterintuitive because the postwar period has seen enormous increases both in overall production and in production per acre. Yet that productivity is directly correlated with the decline he bemoans because the increased yields have come from embracing an industrial model of agriculture that has devastated the land and is not sustainable in the long run.

An industrial model of agriculture comprises an interlocking set of approaches to science, economics, and farming that are yoked together by what Berry describes as an industrial logic. As the logic is applied to agricultural science, it reduces farming to a mere mechanical or chemical process. Economically, industrial logic leads us to treat workers, in this case, farmers, "no different from raw materials or machine parts" (2005, p. 79). Berry writes that promoters of such a view "believe that a farm or a forest is or ought to be the same as a factory; that care is only minimally involved in the use of the land; . . . that for all practical purposes a machine is as good as (or better than) a human; that the industrial standards of production, efficiency, and profitability are the only standards that are necessary; that the topsoil is lifeless and inert; [and] that soil biology is safely replaceable by soil chemistry" (1996, p. 410).

The consequences of treating a farm essentially as a machine are, however, disastrous. Yes, productivity—measured solely as yield per acre—has increased but so, too, have the use of chemicals, the erosion of topsoil, and rates of foreclosures on family farms. Farms have become bigger, less diverse, and so disconnected from local communities—indeed from those who do the work on the farm—that "the result is utterly strange in human experience: farm families who buy everything they eat at the store" (2005, p. 97).

And the industrial model is not confined simply to matters of food production. Berry notes that both farms *and forests* have come to be thought of in industrial or mechanical terms. He also observes the baleful effects of thinking of nature in these reductive terms. The traditional respect, reverence, and awe with which humans approached nature have been lost. In their place, we find a consumerist mindset that sees nature merely as raw material to be used without limit or constraint. "By means of the machine metaphor," Berry writes, "we have eliminated any fear or awe or reverence or humility or delight or joy that might have restrained us in our use of the world" (1986, p. 56). As Berry puts it elsewhere, we grope obsessively and destructively toward the use of everything (1995, p. 2).

If this is Berry's critique of an industrial worldview as it applies to our understanding of nature, what does he suggest as an alternative? Not surprisingly, his model for approaching the natural world is taken from the ideal of an old-fashioned farmer. Berry draws a distinction between someone whose fundamental commitment is to control and maximize short-term productivity with someone whose core value is nurture and sustenance. If the latter is best represented by a traditional farmer, the former is represented by the quintessential exploiter, a strip miner. "The exploiter is a specialist, an expert; the nurturer is not. The standard of the exploiter is efficiency; the standard of the nurturer is care. The exploiter's goal is money, profit; the nurturer's goal is health. . . . Whereas the exploiter asks of a piece of land only how much and how quickly it can be made to produce, the nurturer asks a question that is much more complex and difficult: . . . What can it produce dependably for an indefinite time? . . . The exploiter thinks in terms of numbers, quantities, 'hard facts'; the nurturer is terms of character, condition, quality, kind" (1986, pp. 7–8). Ultimately, Berry believes debates about our conceptions of nature and wilderness are tied to issues of character and its definition. In a chapter in *The Unsettling of America* entitled "The Ecological Crisis as a Crisis of Character," he makes clear that loss of the virtue of self-restraint goes hand-in-glove with an instrumentalist conception of nature as something controlled by us, as if we were not fundamentally a part of nature.

Here we circle back to connect with Cormac McCarthy's view of nature and wilderness set out in the first part of this chapter, for Berry shares with McCarthy an appreciation of the virtue of humility and its relation to conceptions of nature and of wilderness. Indeed, both Berry and McCarthy urge us to a greater sense of respect and reverence for nature. The language of reverence here may suggest that both writers adopt an essentially religious understanding of nature, but drawing that conclusion would, I think, be mistaken. To be sure, some of Berry's writings are explicitly religious, but his defense of a reverential view of nature and its relation to the virtue of humility is not.

We can see this in an essay from *A Continuous Harmony* entitled "A Secular Pilgrimage." In it, Berry turns to poetry to capture what he understands the proper attitude to nature to be. Writing about contemporary poets who turn to nature not just for symbols or metaphors but for subject matter and inspiration, Berry says that "their art has an implicit and essential humility, a reluctance to impose on things as they are, a willingness to relate to the world as student and servant, a wish to be included in the natural order rather than to 'conquer nature'" (1972, p. 4). This attitude requires no institutional religious framework, nor for that matter does it require a belief in god. But it can still be spoken of as a pilgrimage because it involves a quest for meaning that requires us to situate ourselves harmoniously in the world around us.

Once again, there is an instructive parallel with Michael Sandel's position in *The Case against Perfection*. I already noted how Sandel contrasts humility with what he refers to as "hyperagency" and the drive to mastery, and that, in this regard, his vision of the human tendency to disregard limits is similar to Cormac McCarthy's. A closer look at Sandel's argument also sheds light on Wendell Berry's ideas of a "secular pilgrimage." In decrying the "drive to mastery," Sandel articulates what he refers to as an "ethic of giftedness," namely, an ethic that approaches human life as a gift. In developing the idea of the giftedness of human life, Sandel draws on William F. May's notion of an "openness to the unbidden" (2007, p. 45). "May's resonant phrase describes a quality of character and heart that restrains the impulse to mastery and control and prompts a sense of life as gift" (p. 46). The idea that life is a gift, like the notion of a pilgrimage, can be understood in religious terms, but it need not be. As Sandel points out, we frequently speak of an athlete's or a musician's gift without presupposing that the gift came from God (p. 93). Instead, the idea of life as a gift, like the idea of life as a pilgrimage, is meant to combat what he calls the "Promethean ambition to remake nature" (p. 26) and what Berry refers to as technology's "totalitarian desire for absolute control" (1986, p. 130).

Sandel's analysis of an ethic of giftedness, an ethic that requires us to resist the drive to mastery, helps us appreciate how the appeal to nature and wilderness functions for Berry. The key is Sandel's recognition that an ethic of giftedness is reciprocally related to the virtue of humility. An appreciation for the gifted character of human powers and achievements is conducive to the cultivation of humility, and the virtue of humility helps us resist the urge to remake the world (2007, pp. 26–27). The familiar categories of autonomy and rights or calculations of costs and benefits do not exhaust the moral issues at stake; for one thing, these categories are understood too narrowly in individualistic terms. Instead, what is crucial is the "habit of mind and way of being" that an ethic of giftedness seeks to foster (p. 96).

Sandel's language beautifully captures the essence of Berry's view because the industrial worldview Berry decries could well be described as a "habit of mind and a way of being." As we have seen, according to Berry it is a habit of mind that "gropes obsessively and destructively toward the use of everything." And when this worldview is combined with a liberal individualist ethos, the result is a way of being that presupposes a " 'right' of individuals to do as they please, as if there were no God, no legitimate government, no community, no neighbors, and no posterity" (2005, p. 9).

What does Berry offer as an alternative habit of mind and way of being? The answer is put forcefully in a collection of essays whose title, *The Way of Ignorance*, gestures toward Berry's response. This title is intentionally provocative. Berry is not, of course, recommending or praising ignorance; instead, he is commending a way of being that recognizes the limits of our knowledge and the dangers of failing to acknowledge our limits. I would be inclined toward a different formulation of Berry's title, perhaps "the way of mystery" or "the way of wonder," but the essential features of such a worldview would be the same. If an industrial worldview is preoccupied with control and "hyperagency," the way of wonder emphasizes preservation and modesty.

The connection between the way of wonder and wilderness is captured succinctly in Berry's essay "The Journey's End." "Going to the woods and the wild places has little to do with recreation, and much to do with creation. For the wilderness is the creation in its pure state, its processes unqualified by the doings of people. A man in the woods comes face to face with the creation, of which he must begin to see himself a part—a much less imposing part than he thought. And seeing that the creation survives all wishful preconceptions about it, that it includes him only upon its own sovereign terms, that he is not free except in his proper place in it, then he may begin, perhaps, to take a hand in the creation of himself" (1995b, p. 6). Although Berry gets carried away here with his talk of "creation in its pure state," the core idea strikes me as both sound and insightful. Wilderness can help us appreciate nature on its terms rather than ours. "As long as we insist on relating to it strictly on our own terms—as strange to us or subject to us—the wilderness is alien, threatening, fearful. We have no choice then but to become its exploiters, and to lose, by consequence, our place in it. It is only when, by humility, openness, generosity, courage, we make ourselves able to relate to it on its terms that it ceases to be alien" (p. 6).

Nature and Human Overreaching

If we compare Berry's work to McCarthy's, we can see that although there is much they might not agree on, they do have a fundamental commonality of vision. Both recommend cultivating a set of virtues that constrain human overreaching. Both endorse a habit of mind and a way of being in the world that understands and accepts the limits of human knowledge. And both believe that careful attention to nature, and especially to wilderness, promotes what Aldo Leopold referred to as "thinking like a mountain." Such is their mutual vision, but is this vision useful to our project? I believe that it is, but it will not be useful in any easy way because it is more about cultivating certain virtues than about identifying prohibited actions or practices.

We can perhaps better see the complex utility of this vision by examining a recent effort to assess appeals to nature in bioethics. In an essay entitled "Human Nature and Enhancement," Allen Buchanan reviews various appeals to the idea of "human nature" in debates about whether it is morally acceptable to enhance human beings through biotechnology. Buchanan notes that opponents of enhancement technology frequently argue that genetic enhancement will destroy human nature and that destroying or fundamentally changing humans is either per se wrong or wrong because doing so will strip us of the ability to make moral judgments, given that such judgments are tied to a stable conception of human nature.

In evaluating these claims, Buchanan identifies five different forms of the appeal to human nature and argues that all five are fatally flawed. The five forms are human nature understood as (1) a condition of moral agency; (2) a feasibility constraint on morality; (3) a constraint on the good for humans; (4) a source of substantive moral rules; and (5) a complex whole of interdependent characteristics (2009, p. 5). The details of Buchanan's analysis are not crucial for us here. What is crucial is that each kind of appeal is mobilized to suggest either that altering human nature is intrinsically wrong or that doing so will have such disastrous moral consequences that changing our natures is morally prohibited. Buchanan is concerned to demonstrate that appeals to "human nature" cannot ground either of these convictions and are therefore ultimately unhelpful in debates about enhancement.

By way of contrast, the sort of attention to nature and to wilderness that both McCarthy and Berry recommend is not intended to produce concrete guidelines or to support an antitechnology ethos. For example, neither McCarthy nor Berry would find altering human nature intrinsically wrong and neither would necessarily conclude that the consequences of genetically enhancing humans would be so potentially negative that we should categorically prohibit such an action. The closest they come to the positions Buchanan examines is "human nature as a complex whole." According to Buchanan, this form of argument appeals to "nature" to convey a sense of complex and harmonious interdependencies that will be disrupted as humans develop and use biotechnology. But if the appeal to "nature" is a just a shorthand way of acknowledging the "fragility of wholeness," Buchanan says, such appeals are "pernicious" because they encourage "the delusion that reflection on human nature can yield substantive moral rules." Once again, he concludes, "the appeal to human nature is eliminable without loss" (p. 20).

If the goal of appeals to nature is to generate substantive moral rules, then Buchanan is probably right. But, at least in the case of McCarthy and Berry, generating moral rules is not the point of attending to nature and to wilderness. Here, being outside the world of traditional bioethics is probably an asset because these writers are not concerned with generating rules or guidelines. Instead, they recommend attention to nature and wilderness as an exercise that is useful to the development of character. In particular, close attention to nature and personal experience with wilderness are conducive to the development of humility.

The experience of watching a wolf at night in the mountains or plowing a field on a farm during the day is not going to generate a moral calculus for making decisions about the use of biotechnology; Buchanan is right about that. Nevertheless, these kinds of activities can perhaps make us less susceptible to the pull of the Promethean ambition of humans as the masters of the universe. These and similar activities can help us to develop a proper sense of scale; they can remind us of our smallness in the universe; they can foster a sense of awe that may lead us to be more cautious in the use of our powers. Just how attention to nature and wilderness and a corresponding sense of awe and humility can be morally instructive is difficult to say, but let me end by giving an example from Berry's work that might be helpful, in part because it covers some familiar bioethics terrain.

In a superb essay entitled "Quantity vs. Form," Berry recounts the last days of one of his neighbors. "Lily," as he calls her, was suffering from heart disease, osteoporosis, and a bout of pneumonia. In Berry's words, "she was as ill probably as a living creature can be" (2005, p. 82). She was also in great pain. But Lily was reconciled to her death because she had her affairs in order and she judged her life to have been both good and complete. This, says Berry, was something the resident treating her could not understand. Trained in the ways of modern medicine, and thus driven by a technological imperative that typically fails to acknowledge that life can reach an appropriate end and that death can be "a welcome deliverance from pain or grief or weariness" (p. 85), the resident took Lily off her pain medications in the hope of increasing her appetite and getting her back on her feet. To the resident's way of thinking, Lily's death was unnecessary; to Berry's way of thinking, Lily's graceful acceptance of death was deeply admirable.

This example shows the subtle way that the habit of mind and way of being recommended by Berry can apply to difficult moral decisions. If you approach this case in terms of traditional categories of bioethical analysis, you might conclude that Berry is making an argument in favor of euthanasia or assisted suicide. But this is not what he is doing. He is not arguing for a particular position on euthanasia and appealing to nature in a prescriptive way. Instead, he is recommending the development of a more capacious worldview than one that defines medical success in terms of days or weeks of increased longevity. And the support for such a view will not come from principles or norms of bioethics but from an appreciation of limits and genuine humility. Berry puts the point in terms that McCarthy would appreciate. Medicine's preoccupation with extending life expectancy "badly needs a meeting on open ground with tragedy, absurdity, and moral horror" (2005, p. 86). Frequently, that open ground can be found in nature and encounters with wilderness.

What Berry recommends here in thinking about end-of-life issues, he would also recommend for thinking about issues of medical biotechnology, agricultural biotechnology, and environmentalism. The last paragraph of his essay "Local Knowledge in the Age of Information" could well serve as a summary of most of Berry's work, as well as of this chapter: "Our great modern powers of science, technology, and industry are always offering themselves to us with the suggestion that we know enough to use them well, that we are intelligent enough to act without limit in our own behalf. But the evidence is now rapidly mounting against us. By living as we do, in our ignorance and our pride, we are diminishing our world and the possibility of life" (2005, p. 125). The notion of "thinking like a mountain" may seem obscure. But whatever else it means, it certainly involves acknowledging our ignorance and our misplaced pride. The virtue of humility may help us with this acknowledgment, and if McCarthy and Berry are correct, careful attention to nature and wilderness is a good place to begin the cultivation of humility.

NOTES

1. Jacqueline Scoones (2001) has made some interesting connections between McCarthy and Leopold.
2. We learn later that Echols has trapped and killed virtually all of the wolves in this land.
3. On this point, see Arnold (2002).
4. For other examples of Berry's relevant essays on this topic, see 1983, 1984, 1995a, 1999, 2002a, 2002b.

REFERENCES

Arnold, E. T. 2002. "McCarthy and the Sacred: A Reading of *The Crossing*." In *Cormac McCarthy: New Directions,* ed. J. D. Lilley. Albuquerque: University of New Mexico Press.

Berry, W. 1972. *A Continuous Harmony: Essays Cultural and Agricultural.* San Diego: Harcourt Brace Jovanovich.

———. 1983. *Standing by Words.* San Francisco: North Point.

———. 1984. "Whose Head Is the Farmer Using? Whose Head Is Using the Farmer?" In *Meeting the Expectations of the Land: Essays in Sustainable Agriculture and Stewardship,* ed. W. Jackson, W. Berry, and B. Colman, pp. 19–30. San Francisco: North Point.

———. 1986. *The Unsettling of America: Culture and Agriculture.* San Francisco: Sierra Club Books.

———. 1995a. "The Conservation of Nature and the Preservation of Humanity." In *Another Turn of the Crank,* pp. 64–85. Washington, D.C.: Counterpoint.

———. 1995b. "The Journey's End." In *Words from the Land: Encounters with Natural History Writing,* ed. S. Trimble, pp. 226–38. Reno: University of Nevada Press.

———. 1996. "Conserving Communities." In *The Case against the Global Economy: And for a Turn toward the Local,* ed. J. Mander and E. Goldsmith, pp. 407–17. San Francisco: Sierra Club Books.

———. 1999. "The Pleasures of Eating." In *Consumer Society in American History: A Reader,* ed. L. B. Glickman, pp. 367–72. Ithaca, N.Y.: Cornell University Press.

———. 2002a. "Feminism, the Body, and the Machine." In *The Art of the Common-Place,* ed. N. Wirzba, pp. 65–80. Washington, D.C.: Counterpoint.

———. 2002b. "The Idea of a Local Economy." In *The Good in Nature and Humanity: Connecting Science, Religion, and Spirituality with the Natural World,* ed. S. R. Kellert and T. J. Farnham, pp. 199–211. Washington, D.C.: Island Press.

———. 2005. *The Way of Ignorance.* Berkeley, Calif.: Counterpoint.

Buchanan, A. 2009. "Human Nature and Enhancement." *Bioethics* 23 (3): 141–50.

Kaebnick, G. E. 2007. "Putting Concerns about Nature into Context: The Case of Agricultural Biotechnology." *Perspectives in Biology and Medicine* 50 (4): 572–84.

Leopold, A. 2001. *A Sand County Almanac.* New York: Oxford University Press.

McCarthy, C. 1994. *The Crossing.* New York: Alfred A. Knopf.

———. 2006. *The Road.* New York: Alfred A. Knopf.

Sandel, M. J. 2007. *The Case against Perfection: Ethics in the Age of Genetic Engineering.* Cambridge, Mass.: Belknap Press of Harvard University Press.

Scoones, J. 2001. "The World on Fire: Ethics and Evolution in Cormac McCarthy's Border Trilogy." In *A Cormac McCarthy Companion: The Border Trilogy,* ed. E. Arnold and D. Luce, pp. 131–60. Jackson: University Press of Mississippi.

CHAPTER NINE

He Did It on Hot Dogs and Beer

Natural Excellence in Human Athletic Achievement

David Wasserman, J.D., M.A.

There is a great deal of sanctimony in the condemnation of Barry Bonds for allegedly using steroids to acquire the muscle power to break the season and lifetime homerun records once held by Babe Ruth. Had steroids been available, the voracious Babe might have used them with the same abandon with which he consumed hot dogs and beer. But behind the sanctimony lies genuine disappointment that the public cannot take more complete satisfaction in Bonds's prodigious hitting. The claim that he cheated is in one sense about his alleged violation of the rules of the game, which prohibit steroid use. But it is also, perhaps more strongly, about the justification for the rule: even if baseball permitted steroids, those complaining about Bonds would still be inclined to put an asterisk next to his records and would reject the rule as undermining the spirit of the game. Babe Ruth's records, as well as those of Roger Maris and Hank Aaron, are seen as natural human achievements in a way that Bonds's is not. The former achievements realized human potential; the latter do not. But Bonds is obviously human, and the instruments he used to set his records were no more artificial (or more so only to an acceptable extent) than those used by the Sultan of Swat. How can his use of steroids undermine his claim to have more fully realized human potential than his predecessors?

The collective pride we are supposed to take at the unending succession of longer jumps, higher vaults, heavier presses, and so forth is predicated on the notion that relentless competition and steady improvement in nutrition, exercise, and coaching serve to bring us ever closer to realizing our full potential as a species. Paul Weiss articulated a notion of sports as revealing a distinctively human excellence, in which all humans partake, when he declared that "It is because he is an outstanding instance of what man might do and be that an athlete is an outstanding man. . . . Athletes are excellence in the guise of man" (1969, p. 17). For Weiss, athletic achievement redounded to the glory of humanity, not of the individual athlete. But this suggests that the achievement must manifest the latent excellence of human beings—that it must realize a *human* potential.

Human potential can apparently be realized by some sorts of outside intervention, while being superseded or bypassed by others. Muscles can be strengthened by the latest exercise technology but not by drugs; performance can be enhanced by improvement in equipment, such as pole vaults and sneakers, but not by propulsive devices, except in auto racing and the like. An athlete who breaks a record with a fiberglass pole has more fully realized human potential, but an athlete who breaks a record with a fiberglass limb has manifested an excellence that is not entirely human. True, Oscar Pistorius can now compete in Olympic races with a prosthetic limb but only because of a finding that his use of the limbs expends as much energy as a typical athlete's use of his own natural limb (Wollbring, 2008; Camporesi, 2008). If he were to set a world record, there would still be a temptation to place an asterisk beside his name.

The general issue raised by the use of biotechnology to enhance athletic performance can be framed as follows: What would be lost if the pharmacological, medical, or genetic enhancement of athletic performance were (to modify the Clinton slogan about abortion) safe, legal, and widespread? Athletes would certainly train as hard—the legality and the widespread use of biotechnological enhancement would protect enhanced athletes against complacency and lax training. It would be not only dogmatic but also implausible to insist that such changes would inevitably reduce the quality or excitement of competition. Imagine the impact on boxing if most heavyweight contenders could float like butterflies and sting like bees! If biotechnological enhancements will not necessarily dampen the intensity or excitement of athletic competition, however, they may alter other aspects of sports that make them valuable to players and fans. In exploring the anxieties raised by biological enhancement, I seek to identify the values it appears to threaten.

I begin by looking at the more plausible objections proffered by critics of biotechnological enhancement and argue that they fail to justify the categorical exclusion of many enhancements or to provide a clear distinction between the natural and artificial. I then turn to the critique of biological enhancement by the President's Council on Bioethics (2003), which suggests several more credible misgivings about the effects of technological interventions on the meaning and value of athletic competition. These misgivings, however, are not specific, let alone unique, to biotechnology and have greater force for some sports than others. I seek to link these specific misgivings with the more general appeals to nature made in the debates over enhancement in other domains. In connecting the two, I adopt an account that treats such appeals to nature as invocations of the social and cultural background constraints that give meaning to human activities. In the final section, I consider how differences in the background constraints for various sports, and for other important human activities, may bear on the acceptability of biotechnological enhancement.

Some Standard Objections

The primary objection to biotechnological enhancement may not concern the natural condition of the athlete so much as the locus of control or agency for the athletic performance. If an athlete's performance depends on bioengineering, the locus of agency may shift from athlete to engineer, reducing the athlete to a puppet or instrument with little more control over his own performance than a remote-controlled robot. Although this shift may be facilitated by technology, however, it does not require it. Intrusive coaches often achieve victory in a way that is perceived as diminishing the achievement of the athlete or team. Moreover, this concern about agency cannot explain the rejection of many "internal improvements," from prostheses to steroids, that do not reduce an athlete's own control of his training and performance, though they may alter how he trains or performs. The growing number of tactical decisions made by coaches and trainers, in sports ranging from basketball to boxing, represents a much greater threat to the agency of individual athletes.

The concern for realizing and preserving fully human potential thus appears to be more about authenticity than control, about improvements that alter the human body regardless of their effect on agency. No artifice compromises the body if it is sufficiently external to it. A fiberglass pole is not natural; it is only an instrument that a natural body can use with varying degrees of proficiency. In contrast, a prosthesis or steroid injection might be thought to render the body unnatural. Of course, we are all adulterated to some extent by human intervention—the content of our diet has been radically altered by agricultural biotechnology, and our bones, teeth, and organs bear the imprint, and often the residues of medical intervention. One obvious concern is that an athlete with extensive germ-line or even somatic genetic modifications would no longer be human (and therefore not the same individual, on some views of personal identity). Clearly, a transhuman or posthuman champion would not be "an outstanding instance of what man might do and be" (Weiss, 1969, p. 17). But although genetic engineering raises challenges for the definition of "species" and the boundaries between species, the kind of genetic enhancements contemplated for athletes would be unlikely to place them outside any plausible species boundaries.

Nor will a gradualist objection to pharmacological and genetic enhancement work here—the claim that biotechnology is objectionable simply because it would further denature athletes and athletic performance. We do not think that the contemporary athletes who benefit from the best scientific nutrition and training are less natural, in any sense that we care about, than the hot-dog snarfing, beer-swilling athletes of yore, just more fortunate and advantaged. At least here, there seems to be no slippery slope to descend. While some writers on the idea of nature suggest that the human impact on the landscape became "unnatural" with the advent of the industrial revolution (see Soper, 1995), we do not seem to have an analogous sense about the impact of training technology on athletes' bodies, a sense of when a difference in degree becomes a difference in kind. If there is a plausible concern about the metamorphosis of the human body into an artifice, it is not raised by steroids but by prosthetics. There may well be compelling reasons for the International Olympic Committee's decision to admit Oscar Pistorius to Olympic competition. But if a runner can compete with one prosthetic limb, then why not with two, or four? (See Wollbring, 2008; Camporesi, 2008.) A gold medal won with four prosthetic limbs might celebrate human excellence, but it arguably would not celebrate the excellence of the human body. The ingestion of steroids, however, does not make the athlete's body any less human than the ingestion of other substances.

There may also be a concern that steroid use may threaten the natural hierarchy that sports celebrate (Juengst, 2009). But unlike the advent of firearms, which appeared to threaten the hierarchy of martial prowess that evolved in an age of jousting and swordplay, there is no reason to think that legal steroid use will level, or even broaden, the hierarchy of athletic performance. It may cause significant changes as to where individual athletes fall within that hierarchy, but so have many other changes in sports. Moreover, the extent to which it will do so and the identity of those it will affect are uncertain.

Finally, there is the matter of what constitutes a "natural process." Why is the injection of steroids not a natural process when the ingestion of protein-rich food is? It cannot be a matter of intent. The intent in taking steroids may be to build bulk, but the protein supplements sold in health and sports stores are bought with the same intent. We accept as natural supplying the genome with outside nutrients—we could hardly exist if we did not. We accept as natural varying the mix of nutrients for specific purposes—bulking up for a long winter or a big mastodon hunt. But injecting refined chemicals into the bloodstream we reject. Yet it is not unnatural, or not objectionably so, for athletes to have shots for therapeutic purposes. This suggests a notion of purity in-the-alternative: if the substances an athlete takes are impure, like most medicines, then that athlete's motives must be pure—that is, therapeutic. If the substances are pure, however, like "natural" protein supplements, then his motives need not be pure. This may be a partial explanation of our discomfort with biotechnological enhancement, but it seems hopeless as a justification.

The elusive notion of natural process also plays a central role in the controversy over low-oxygen training. Long-distance runners who grew up in high altitudes enjoy an advantage in endurance at lower altitudes, an advantage their lowland competitors have long sought to offset by sleeping at high elevations. Technology has made this advantage more widely available with the development of hypoxic tents, which can boost endurance without the considerable cost and inconvenience of training low and resting high. In a controversial decision, the World Anti-Doping Agency (WADA) proposed banning these tents for athletic training, on the ground that they represent a passive rather than active use of technology to boost athletic performance. The decision was based on the belief that training at high altitudes required more exertion than using low-altitude tents, in which the athlete mainly sleeps (World Anti-Doping Agency, 2006). Although the distinction between active and passive seems a "natural" one for athletic training, critics argued that other accepted enhancements were no less passive. They countered WADA's distinction with the more familiar one between environmental and bodily modification, arguing that athletes have always modified the atmosphere they lived and trained in for comfort and performance (Saletan, 2006; Wallace, 2006). The atmosphere of a hypoxic tent or mask may be a micro- rather than macro-environment, but that struck critics as an irrelevant difference.

WADA and its critics rely on different notions of natural conditioning.[1] The disagreement in this case is not over where the line falls between acceptable and unacceptable conditioning but over what the relevant dimension is: active-passive or external-internal. This suggests that our intuitions about what is natural in the cultivation and enhancement of athletic ability are not just vague but conflicting, providing an unstable basis for any analysis of what qualifies as "natural" in sports.

The Council Weighs In

In *Beyond Therapy* (2003) the President's Council on Bioethics addressed concerns about the meaning and significance of the concept of "the natural" with considerable nuance. It recognized that athletics has long relied on artifice, such as equipment and training, and that the line between acceptable (graphite tennis rackets) and unacceptable (corked bats) innovations was often based on convention and sport-specific. It also acknowledged that improvements in nutrition and training have significantly modified athletes' bodies. But even though biotechnological interventions may differ only in degree from more familiar measures, that does not exempt them from concern: "*the ethical evaluation of biological enhancements does not finally depend on their being found utterly unique and unprecedented*" (p. 124, italics in original). Biotechnology may accelerate existing trends, such as the increasing physical differences and social distance between athletes and fans or the ever more narrow and obsessive character of athletic pursuits.

Yet it is not clear that every trend the President's Council observed is disturbing. Training, in which our experience and self-understanding are aligned, is admittedly different from "interventions that bypass human experience to work their biological 'magic' directly—from nutrition to steroids to genetic muscle enhancement," where "our bodily workings and our conscious agency are more alienated from each other" (p. 130). Yet no one sees improved nutrition as estranging athletes from their bodies or their performance, even when the nutrition is part of a special, performing-enhancing regimen.[2] The fact that nutrition is beyond our conscious agency hardly alienates us from our bodies; much of the activity necessary for survival and agency, like heartbeat or peristalsis, is outside our control and often our awareness. The bypass of our agency in many strength-enhancing physiological functions is familiar and innocent, not a problematic trend that drug use can be condemned for accelerating. If steroids and genetic muscle enhancement alienate the athlete from his body, it must be because of something they do not share with nutrition.

The council also suggested that biotechnological enhancement, unlike better nutrition, contributes to the estrangement of human athletes from their increasingly nonhuman bodies: "The runner on steroids or with genetically enhanced muscles is still, of course, a human being who runs. But the doer of the deed is, arguably, less obviously himself and less obviously human than his unaltered counterpart. He may be faster, but he may also be on the way to becoming 'more cheetah' than man, or more like the horse we breed for the race-track than a self-willing, self-directed, human agent. He does the deed (running), and his resulting time may be measurably superior. But he is also (or increasingly) the recipient of outside agents that are at least partly responsible for his achievements" (p. 144). "In trying to achieve better bodies through muscle-enhancing agents, pharmacological or genetic, we are not in fact honoring our bodies or cultivating our individual gifts. We are instead, whether we realize it or not, voting with our syringes to have a different body, with different native capacities and powers. We are giving ourselves new and foreign gifts—not nature's, and not our own—exaggerating, but in the direction of the truth, treating ourselves rather as if we were batting machines to be perfected or as superior horses bred for the race and bound to do our bidding" (p. 149).

These concerns may appear little more than an eloquent paraphrase of some of the objections already mentioned. The President's Council seems worried about the loss of agency resulting from biotechnological enhancement, the reduction of a human runner to a racehorse or batting machine. Such concern is misplaced; as noted, there is no reason to think that biotechnology will shift the locus of control away from an athlete any more than intensive coaching does; greater technological assistance need not mean reduced agency.

The real concern in these passages is over authenticity and self-alienation. Because the agent gives himself a "new and foreign gift"—a "different body, with different native capacities and powers"—his performance, however fully under his control, will not really be *his*. He may still be in control, but not of his own natural body. He will be "on the way" to riding a horse or operating a batting machine. Because "he" is both the agent and the object of the agent's will, his self-movement will become divided and opaque, lacking the unity of mind and body found in a natural athlete. The estrangement may ultimately be as profound as, if far more functional than, that experienced by Gregor Samsa upon awakening in the body of a giant insect.

We can agree that a body becomes less natural, in an intuitive sense, when shaped by steroids or genetic engineering, just as it does when its original parts are replaced by prostheses. But there is no reason in principle why these modifications should estrange the agent from his body as Samsa's metamorphosis does to him. Such estrangement would be evidence that the modification was flawed or incomplete. An accident victim who cannot control an artificial limb with the ease or grace with which he controls a natural limb needs a better prosthesis or more practice. Steroids and genetic muscle enhancement would not boost performance if they offered the athlete something akin to a clumsy prosthesis; they would only work if the changes they brought became "second nature." Even if the modified body parts never became the athlete's own in all respects (for example, if they were less sensitive to a breeze or a caress), the athlete could master them in a way that conferred a temporary unity, like a champion vaulter with his pole, a driver with his car, or a jockey with his horse. (Indeed, highly adept and experienced equestrians are sometimes described as "centaurs.")

These adaptations suggest a subtle (or not-so-subtle) modification in the character of the athlete's agency, but they need not result in his alienation or debasement. The problem is not one of degree, as the council suggests, because there is no trend toward mind-body estrangement for steroids to accelerate. The council seems to be doing no more than asserting that an athlete's modified body is alien to him just because it is less natural or less human in a biological sense.

There are, however, more sympathetic interpretations of the council's misgivings. At least three other concerns are suggested by the quoted passages and articulated elsewhere in the report. The first is that injecting steroids or inserting genes involves the repudiation rather than the loving improvement of the athlete's body. The second is that biotechnology will widen the divide between elite athletes and their fans, further attenuating the identification of spectator with player that has been so important to the experience of many sports. The third concern is that the pace and magnitude of the changes biotechnology introduces will drastically alter the character of particular sports, disrupting the continuity between past and present that has been an integral part of those sports for both players and spectators. The second and third concerns are more plausible than the first because they see the risk of biotechnology lying in its contribution to trends that are already undermining or corrupting cherished practices and traditions.

If the President's Council is right, it is no defense that the changes wrought by biotechnology are only a matter of degree. Why should we accept interventions that make valuable practices incrementally worse? Even if the council's concerns are exaggerated—and I will contend that they are—they provide insight into the value of athletic competition and its vulnerability to rapid and comprehensive change. The more plausible of the council's concerns reflect a conception of nature as a set of constraints on human activity that give it meaning and significance. But those constraints vary greatly among different activities, and objections to the erosion of those constraints may lack the generality to which the council aspires.

Repudiation and Ingratitude

The President's Council's concern about the repudiation of the athlete's body is less about the effects of the enhancement than its motivation. Frustrated with the limitations of her natural body, impatient with the modest improvements she can achieve through training and diet, the athlete opts to radically change her body. She is like a parent who tires of instruction and discipline and medicates his rambunctious child or an actor who gives up on cosmetics and undergoes cosmetic surgery. If the use of steroids or gene replacement did manifest such a rejection of "the given," it might well be problematic. But how problematic it was would depend on what it repudiated. To subject one's child to psychopharmacology because one finds him incorrigible may be more problematic than to submit to the knife because one despairs of one's looks. The council talks with insufficient discrimination about the importance of "accepting the given"; unless one regards one's child and one's body as equally gifts from God, there is a stronger moral imperative to accept the former than the latter. To adopt Erik Parens's terms (2005), gratitude may be the dominant framework in parenthood, creativity in athletics.

But there is a more basic problem with the council's concern about repudiation. The presumption that injecting steroids or replacing genes involves a fuller repudiation of one's body than do relentless, punishing training or harsh dietary regimens requires a certain view of what is essential to one's body. A man who spends hours every day at the make-up table, bitterly fretting over his recalcitrant features, may be expressing more self-loathing than a man who gamely undertakes cosmetic surgery to advance his career as a model or soap opera star. Because steroids and gene replacement may be riskier or more harmful than conventional enhancements, it may be reasonable to suppose that their use involves greater repudiation, more desperate competitiveness, or both. But without that risk, the distinction rests on two assumptions the council never defends: (1) that steroid injections and gene replacement are categorically greater changes than conventional enhancements because they alter what is essential to our bodies; (2) that those who would use biotechnological enhancements accept this distinction. Such a combination of undefended metaphysical claims and speculative psychological ones is all too characteristic of the council's work.

The Estrangement of Athletes from Fans

The second concern is about the athlete's estrangement from her fans, not her body, and it has a good deal more plausibility. One powerful motif in American sports legends is that the great athlete is one of us: growing up in the same neighborhood, attending the same school, sharing the same tribulations, engaging in the same transgressions, and even after success and celebrity, keeping the same friends and frequenting the same haunts. It is no Horatio Alger story, suggesting that any of us could have been that star; it is rather, about the extraordinary as ordinary, having enough commonalities with the rest of us to sustain intense identification in the face of surpassing excellence. To proclaim that Babe Ruth did it on hot dogs and beer is to assert not only that he did it without cheating, but also that he did it while eating and looking like us (or even worse). Of course, similarity and identification come in degrees. As Michael Sandel observes, we admire both the hard work and relentless striving of the modestly talented Pete Rose and the effortless grace of the gifted Joe DiMaggio (Sandel, 2004). But while we may identify more strongly with the Pete Roses than the Joe DiMaggios, even those athletes we admire for their awesome talent have well-publicized frailties and limitations that provide a foothold for our identification.

At the same time, our commonality with sports heroes has always been exaggerated. The myth of that commonality that becomes increasing difficult to sustain as sports stars become part of a social and economic, as well as athletic, elite. And it is even harder when athletes come to look less like the rest of us. The extraordinary talent of Ted Williams—"the Splendid Splinter"—was not obvious from his physique. There is something thrilling in the realization that one of baseball's greatest hitters looked more like the proverbial ninety-seven-pound weakling than an Olympic god. There is no similar surprise in looking at Barry Bonds. When stars no longer look like us, live like us, or even talk to us, it may be harder to identify with them or to take vicarious satisfaction in their success. No doubt steroids and gene replacement will make them resemble us even less. As Dr. Theodore Friedman lamented in his testimony to the President's Council about biotechnology and sports enhancement: "I think one has to have faith in one's idols. When I was growing up, I lived just down the street from the Philadelphia Phillies player who was one of the neighbors and just another person. He was an athlete, but he was another one of us. I must say that in watching . . . baseball games, I no longer know what I am seeing. In a way, I feel a little robbed by not really having faith, not as much faith, as I had in my old idol, of the reality that I am now seeing bioengineering . . . and pharmacology more than I am sport."

It is easy to share Friedman's regret that the star player is no longer a neighbor, no longer "just another person." Admittedly, this is a matter of degree, and the social and economic separation of athletes may matter as much or more than their increasing physical differences. Indeed, other commonalities between star athletes and their fans may make the identification of the latter with the former resilient against, if not downright impervious to, fairly radical bodily changes. There was nothing muted about the excitement of local San Francisco fans for Bonds's record-breaking home run, and the public and media hostility toward his achievement may have less to do with his aloof attitude than his outsize physique.

Broken Records and Discontinuity

The concern about records may not rest on the perceived importance of the genome or on the comparative artificiality of steroids but, as the President's Council suggests, on the perceived magnitude and pace of genetic and pharmacological improvements. Dietary change produces improved performance gradually; as the Olympic motto makes clear, we expect our records to be broken again and again. But some may fear that if steroid use were legal and almost-universal among athletes, and medically supervised for maximum effects, past records would be no challenge for most competitors. Steroids would trivialize the past, not honor it in the way that gradual, hard-won record-breaking does. This fear may be reflected in public response to the new home run records. Babe Ruth's single-season record held for over thirty years and finally fell, to intense if bittersweet acclaim, to one player by one home run (in a longer season). Thirty-seven years after that, that record, in turn, fell to two players in one season, by nine runs, and it was broken again a few years later. The sudden, dramatic escalation in home run hitting raises the specter of change so rapid that it threatens to shrink the role of past achievement in the appreciation of present performance.

Yet baseball was as radically transformed by the regular replacement of game balls as it is likely to be by unfettered biological enhancement. Before that change, batters had to hit a dirty, misshapen ball for most of the game. The home run record was twenty-seven, set in 1884. Less than two years after the change, in 1920, Babe Ruth hit fifty-four home runs. The impact of the change was hardly limited to home runs. According to some commentators, the whole nature of the sport was transformed. The game of sly tactical ingenuity epitomized by Ty Cobb was replaced by a competition of powerhouse hitting against high-velocity pitching. Baseball absorbed these changes without a significant loss of continuity or popularity. It has remained the same game, even to the point where recent years have supposedly seen the resurgence of tactical ball over powerhouse hitting (Ward and Burns, 1994).

If we regard both Ty Cobb and Babe Ruth as among baseball's greatest players, recognizing that their achievements are in an important way incommensurable, is it not possible that future generations will make similarly qualified comparisons between Ruth and Bonds? Steroid use could become another one of the changes—like the enlargement of the season and the introduction of the designated hitter—adduced in the vociferous debates on sports-fan radio about the comparative excellence of players and teams in different eras.

The capacity of sports to absorb significant changes does not mean, of course, that those changes are always for the best. Some sports have undoubtedly been changed for the worse, and the legalized use and regulation of steroids might well make baseball a less subtle and artful game. So there may be good reason to "proceed with caution" in accepting biotechnological modifications of athletes even when they are proven safe. But these are practical concerns that invite empirical assessment and a pragmatic response.

The Ideal of the Natural: Conventional, Not Metaphysical?

Even if fears of the President's Council about identification and continuity are exaggerated, they are legitimate concerns. They reinforce the council's point that "the ethical evaluation of biological enhancements does not finally depend on their being found utterly unique and unprecedented" (President's Council, 2003, p. 124). The fact that identification may be attenuated by economic and social factors as well as biological alterations does not make those alterations an insignificant threat. The resilience of sports in the face of significant changes—in the athletes, their equipment, and the rules—has limits. Too many changes too quickly may not merely coarsen a sport or reduce its popularity, but diminish its value for its most devoted performers and observers. And biotechnological enhancement raises the specter of rapid change.

The pace of athletic enhancement is likely to increase dramatically if it is tied to biotechnology because the pace of biotechnological innovation is so rapid. There may be no categorical distinction between the calculated improvement of athletes' diets over the past several centuries and the current development of performance-enhancing drugs, but differences in degree, if sufficiently large, can become differences in kind. The pace of biotechnological innovation may overcome the capacity of a sports culture to integrate it.

Moreover, the changes wrought by biotechnology may be far harder for the sports community to assess on a case-by-case basis. There are still intense debates among baseball players and observers about the impact of the designated hitter on the style and strategy of play, and there were doubtless similar debates about the introduction of ever-livelier balls. Though some effects of some biotechnological enhancements may be highly salient, like faster pitches, longer hits, and more home runs, others may be subtler and more difficult to monitor, like those from technologies that slow muscle exhaustion. It may be more difficult to have informed public debates about those changes than about changes in rules and equipment. This lack of transparency, however innocent, in some of the changes produced by biotechnology, may further alienate performers and spectators from their sports.

Is there any way to link these concerns with the appeals to nature that pervade so many critiques of biological enhancement? Clearly, the more credible anxieties are not about crossing lines between the natural and artificial or turning athletes into machines. Yet if we take seriously Edmund Burke's claim that "art is man's nature" (1791), we may still have grounds for objecting to some kinds of human intervention as "unnatural."

One promising approach understands appeals to nature as appeals to the constraints on choice necessary to confer meaning on human activity. Drawing on earlier work by Richard Norman (1996), Stephen Holland (2003) argues that our achievements must be understood against a backdrop of constraints that arise from cultural "glosses" on brute biological facts about our mortality, vulnerabilities, and limited capacities: "We achieve significance in our choices and actions only when they are made against a backdrop of constraints that are not open to choice. These background conditions comprise facts—about such things as birth, illness, and death—made up of culturally specific glosses. . . . Some practices or procedures apparently threaten to disrupt those background conditions. In that event, our response to those practices or procedures will be hostile; understandably, given the role of the backdrop as necessary conditions for significant choice. . . . One expression of that hostility is the complaint, 'It's unnatural'" (p. 155).

Holland illustrates this account with the example of a runner objecting to a speed-enhancing moveable track on the grounds that it is unnatural. Although the purpose of his training and dietary regiment is to increase his speed, one of the critical constraints on his endeavor is a stationary running surface. A moveable track would deny significance to his actions by removing that constraint. But although the activity of competitive running derives its significance from biological limits on human mobility, the specific constraints that apply to the activity are dictated by convention: "If [runners] run quickly because the track moves, of course, they're cheating; but if they do so because wind moves in a favourable direction, they might still consider it an achievement. Such ambiguities abound. . . . Only certain kinds of equipment are allowable: for example, good running shoes are fine, but a moving track is not. But whatever the anomalies, there's a threshold for defining a background of conditions necessary if their actions are to have significance; if their performance is to count as an achievement" (2003, p. 156).

Although such constraints are in this sense conventional, they cease to be arbitrary once they have been widely accepted and well established. Significant changes can threaten our shared understanding of the meaning of valuable human activities. Equally important, however, it may often be debatable whether they do. As Holland observes, "the debate typically unfolds between conservatives, who see an innovation as a serious threat to supposedly fixed conditions, and liberals, who think it is not a serious threat to the possibility of achievement and significant action" (2003, p. 157). Such debates are not entirely empirical; they pit strict and broad constructions of important cultural practices against one another.

Holland's approach differs in two critical respects from that adopted by the President's Council and other critics of pharmacological and genetic enhancement. First, it does not rest on an opposition between the natural and the artificial. The background constraints that give meaning to human activity are natural in the sense that they are a given for the agent, unchosen and usually unquestioned; they are artificial in the sense that they are a product of the agent's society and culture.

Second, the constraints differ significantly among sports. They differ not only in the trivial sense that different sports have different rules, but to the extent that they serve to limit modifications of the performers' bodies or physical capacities.

Some sports are, in Sigmund Loland's terms, more "vulnerable" to the biotechnology enhancement of their performers than others (2005). Individual sports like track and field, where success depends on a specialized individual skill, are more vulnerable to such enhancements than team sports in which success rests on a mix of physical and mental skills, as well as group dynamics and coordination. The more vulnerable the sport, the less acceptable biotechnological modification is likely to be, and the more of a premium is likely to be placed on keeping the athletes in "a natural state." But even sports that are not as vulnerable overall, like baseball, contain specific activities, such as pitching and hitting, that are. The violation of constraints on bodily enhancement matters more for pitching and hitting than for fielding not only because these are higher-profile activities but because people perceive biotechnological enhancement as more threatening to the meaning and value of individual achievements than to coordinated team activities like fielding.

From Recreation to Procreation: The Generality of a Constraint-Based Account of Appeals to Nature

It is not clear whether the background-constraint account of appeals to nature in sports can fully explain the perceived threat of biotechnology in the domain of athletic competition. Critics like the Presidents' Council on Biotechnology understand the threat as part of a much broader challenge to human dignity and flourishing. The council's case against the pharmacological and genetic enhancement of athletes is hardly the parochial complaint of disgruntled sports fans about changes to familiar conventions; it is part of a more general concern about the alienating and corrupting effects of biotechnology. Although the council would agree that the lines drawn to limit the uses of biotechnology may be arbitrary or conventional, it sees those lines as barriers against the subversion of fundamental human values. For the council, the objection to steroid or gene doping as unnatural has a close kinship to the objections to general cognitive enhancement or reproductive cloning as unnatural. Do accounts of appeals to nature in terms of background constraints on human activity have the resources to explain this connection, or must they reject it as superficial or exaggerated?

One response to the council is that its understanding of nature is too rigid. "Nature" is a fuzzy concept; it lacks a core meaning that holds constant across the range of contexts in which it is employed. Thus, Gregory Kaebnick argues that "claims about the value of nature also depend partly on claims about the value of concepts. Many perfectly serviceable concepts often are—and must be—delineated only loosely" (2007, p. 577). The "fuzziness" of concepts complicates their application: "We will have to consider how nature is used in different domains—in debates about agriculture, the environment, and human nature—and probably also within specific contexts within those broad domains. . . . Within the debate on human nature, we may find that considerations about enhancement differ depending on context. We may find that what counts as 'natural' is unproblematic in some cases, contestable in others, and too indeterminate to be of any use in others" (p. 578).

Kaebnick suggests that we might regard claims about what is natural as "important and defensible in debates about sports doping (perhaps arguing that athletic competition is to test and celebrate natural human activities as developed and refined through training and discipline)" (p. 578). But even in that context, the truth of such claims may be indeterminate: "If an athlete sleeps in a low-pressure tent, is the athlete 'doping'? Arguments can likely be made one way and the other, with no great likelihood of settling the matter. Still other cases may lead themselves reasonably well to some one understanding of how the concepts apply, yet still remain *under*determined: an athlete who takes testosterone because of a testicular malfunction is probably not doping—but how can we be sure?" (pp. 577–78). Kaebnick does not discuss how the concept of "human nature" applies in other domains addressed by the President's Council, such as genetic enhancement and cloning. But his analysis leaves open the possibility that talk of nature in these domains may be "too indeterminate to be of any use."

Yet the background-constraints account of appeals to nature may prove useful in finding commonalities in appeals to nature across domains, not in the specific constraints that are imposed or invoked, but in the common need to confer and preserve the meaning of the activities in these domains. Indeed, while Holland uses sports to illustrate his account, he actually applies it to three areas of reproductive technology: artificial reproduction, genetic enhancement, and human cloning. In each context, he identifies distinct constraints that appear to be threatened by biotechnology: the connection between sex and procreation in assisted reproduction; the nurturing role of parents in genetic enhancement; both of these in human cloning. He does not argue either for the value of the constraint—many people regard sex and procreation as well severed—or for the reality of the perceived threat—genetically enhanced children may pose greater nurturing challenges for their parents than unenhanced children. His point is rather that debates about whether various biotechnological interventions are "unnatural" are really about the value and the frailty of the constraints they appear to threaten.

Of course, the background constraints for sports and human reproduction differ profoundly, and comparing the two may seem to trivialize the latter. The debasement of a sport whose constraints get swept away by reckless innovation (a fate some believe to have befallen power lifting; see Todd and Todd, 2009) is a misfortune. The divorce of procreation from adult love, or of child development from parental nurturing, would be a tragedy. Moreover, there are always other sports that have not been debased, or are more resistant to debasement, but there are few socially viable options for creating and rearing children. There seems no reason, however, why this vast difference in the magnitude of the loss should make the use of a constraints analysis inapt in either domain.

If anything, a comparison of background constraints in the two domains may be a source of insight into both. The comparison may indicate that there is greater resilience and flexibility in one or both than is commonly assumed. The desire to test one's physical limits against others similarly engaged can be fulfilled by indefinitely many forms of athletic competition; a variety of practices may ensure that the creation and nurturing of children can be achieved within the most intimate relationships. The comparison may also suggest that the same desires and values the constraints protect are a threat to these constraints. The competitive urge often threatens the constraints on competition that make its expression meaningful; the yearning to have and to rear children may not respect age, partnership, or other eligibility conditions that make the creation and rearing of children a meaningful practice.

Let me return to the question with which I began this chapter: what would be lost if the pharmacological, medical, or genetic enhancement of athletic performance were safe, legal, and widespread? The short answer is that we do not know. The present illegality of performance-enhancing drugs, however justifiable, has precluded efforts to accommodate the use of those drugs within any sport—with the notable exception of power lifting. The experience of that sport—a proliferation of leagues with ill-defined and ill-enforced rules—is not encouraging, but it is also not representative (Todd and Todd, 2009). Power lifting is not only a highly vulnerable sport—pharmacological enhancement has a direct and substantial impact on the entire performance—but also a notably fractious one, tending to attract convention-disdaining mavericks. A sport like baseball, less vulnerable and at least outwardly more respectful of rules and traditions, might be more likely to accommodate performance-enhancing drugs "internally," with limits on use and, perhaps, the kind of "positional segregation" that the sport is now accused of engaging in racially—coaches might be expected or encouraged to place their enhanced players in the outfield rather than on the pitcher's mound. What is clear is that we cannot predict the specific accommodations that would be made or how they would affect, and be perceived as affecting, the character of the sport. Despite our wholesale uncertainty, however, it is important to recognize that surrender to performance-enhancing drugs need not be unconditional. We may have the resources to develop conventions and practices that may eventually make some forms of doping more "natural" than others.

NOTES

1. Neither side in the hypoxic tent controversy has relied on the intent with which the environment is modified. The intent to enhance is as specific for athletes who bring themselves to the mountain as it is for athletes who bring the mountain to them.

2. Wheaties was called the "the breakfast of champions" because it supposedly contained nutrients that were unavailable in such concentrated forms to the athletes of past generations.

REFERENCES

Burke, E. 1791. "Letter from the New to the Old Whigs." www.ourcivilization.com/smartboard/shop/burke/extracts/chap17.htm.

Camporesi, S. 2008. "Oscar Pistorius, Enhancement, and Post-Humans." *Journal of Medical Ethics* 34:639.

Holland, S. 2003. *Bioethics: A Philosophical Introduction.* Cambridge, U.K.: Polity.

Juengst, E. T. 2009. "Annotating the Moral Map of Enhancement: Gene Doping, the Limits of Medicine, and the Spirit of Sport." In *Performance-Enhancing Technologies in Sports: Ethical, Conceptual and Scientific Issues,* ed. T. H. Murray, K. J. Maschke, and A. A. Wasunna. Baltimore: Johns Hopkins University Press.

Kaebnick, G. E. 2007. "Putting Concerns about Nature in Context: The Case of Agricultural Biotechnology." *Perspectives in Biology and Medicine* 50 (4): 572–84.

Loland, S. 2005. "The Vulnerability Thesis and the Use of Bio-Medical Technology in Sport." In *Genetic Technology and Sport: Ethical Questions,* ed. C. Tamburrini and T. Tännsjö, pp. 158–64. New York: Routledge.

Norman, R. 1996. "Interfering with Nature." *Journal of Applied Philosophy* 13:1–11.

Parens, E. 2005. "Authenticity and Ambivalence: Towards Understanding the Enhancement Debate." *Hastings Center Report* 35 (3): 34–41.

President's Council on Bioethics. 2003. *Beyond Therapy: Biotechnology and the Pursuit of Happiness*. Washington, D.C.

Sandel, M. 2004. "The Case against Perfection: What's Wrong with Designer Children, Bionic Athletes, and Genetic Engineering." *Atlantic Monthly*, April.

Soper, K. 1995. *What Is Nature?* Oxford: Blackwell.

Todd, J., and T. Todd. 2009. "Reflections on the 'Parallel Federal Solution' to the Problem of Drug Use in Sport: The Cautionary Tale of Powerlifting." In *Performance-Enhancing Technologies in Sports: Ethical, Conceptual and Scientific Issues*, ed. T. H. Murray, K. J. Maschke, and A. A. Wasunna. Baltimore: Johns Hopkins University Press.

Wallace, S. "Why WADA Has It Wrong on Simulated Altitude Systems." www.altitude forall.info/hypoxia_resources_wallace1.html (accessed October 5, 2006).

Ward, G. C., and K. Burns. 1994. *Baseball: An Illustrated History*. New York: Knopf.

Weiss, P. 1969. *Sport: A Philosophical Inquiry*. Carbondale: Southern Illinois University Press.

Wollbring, G. 2008. "Oscar Pistorius and the Future Nature of Olympic, Paralympic and Other Sports." *SCRIPTed* 5 (1). www.law.ed.ac.uk/ahrc/script-ed/vol5-1/wolbring .asp.

World Anti-Doping Agency. 2006. "WADA Note on Artificially-Induced Hypoxic Conditions." www.wada-ama.org/rtecotent/document.

CHAPTER TEN

Sport, Simulation, and EPO

Nicholas Agar, Ph.D.

This chapter addresses the morality of performance-enhancing drugs and modifications in sport. It is motivated by the belief that the decisions we as a public make about cyclists injecting synthetic EPO and weightlifters using genetic technology to make their muscles bigger will act as powerful moral precedents for the more dramatic revisions of human nature that may soon come.

A variety of drugs and modifications can justifiably be excluded from elite sport. The interests of spectators are key to this exclusion. Put simply, spectators want to watch sporting performances that are not only exceptional but also produced by competitors similar to them in ways they care about. Performance-enhancing drugs and genetic modifications offend against this interest. This is what justifies banning them.

Two Spectator Interests in Elite Sport

There are many differences between elite sports and the amateur variety many people practice on Saturday mornings. One key difference is the presence of audiences. Elite sporting events are performances that could not exist in anything like their current form without audiences. Gone would be the endorsements, advertising revenues, cable TV subscriptions, and ticket sales that support elite sportspeople and their retinues. If sport is a performance provided for spectators, then it seems appropriate to emphasize their interests. It is reasonable to ask what exactly we are paying for.

A significant spectator interest directs against many performance-enhancing measures. Among measures that conflict with this interest are injections of the synthetic version of erythropoietin (EPO) that boost the oxygen-carrying capacity of blood; anabolic steroids that increase the capacity to train; certain stimulants that increase alertness, competitiveness, and aggression; and a variety of modifications of genetic material that may provide competitive advantage. Such a spectator interest justifies the current regulatory regime of the World Anti-Doping Agency (WADA).

That spectators' needs justify restrictions on enhancements may be a surprising conclusion to those who attribute the proliferation of banned enhancers in elite sport to an audience demand for ever more extreme performances.[1] Sport lies at the intersection of a variety of sometimes conflicting interests, some of which are compatible with, or even require, enhancement. We have an *interest in extremes*. We watch telecasts of the fastest humans with some of the same zeal that we watch documentaries about the deepest-diving sea mammals and about the migratory birds that fly the farthest. Performance-enhancing measures are not only compatible with this interest, they promote it.

Many of the measures banned by WADA are incompatible, however, with an *interest in identifying*. When we watch sport we have the opportunity to experience exceptional performances "from the inside." When the interest in identifying and the interest in extremes come into conflict, watchers of sport judge identification to be more important. Its priority among our values explains many of the judgments we make about sport. The interest in identifying generates our harsh assessments of those caught doping and the widespread disaffection with sports in which doping seems to be widespread.

McKibben on the Tedium of Enhanced Marathons

How might performance enhancers disappoint spectators? In his book *Enough*, Bill McKibben argues against the performance enhancements made possible by modifying marathoners' genomes. He thinks that such enhancements would make marathons plain boring. According to McKibben, if marathoners genetically enhance themselves, "we won't just lose races, we'll lose racing: we'll lose the possibility of the test, the challenge, the celebration that athletics represents" (2003, pp. 6–7). This is because genetic enhancement transforms the marathon from an event in which competitors are pushed to their physical and mental limits into one in which they perform according to their design specifications. McKibben says that running would become "like driving." He allows that "driving can be fun" but insists that "the skill, the engagement, the meaning reside mostly in those who design the machines" (pp. 6–7). This last claim might be news to Michael Schumacher.

The suggestion that there will be no challenges for genetically modified athletes confuses enhancement with omnipotence. Of course there will be challenges for genetically enhanced athletes. If we allow genetic enhancement, we won't "lose racing." We may lose some of the races that humans currently compete in. If 42.195 kilometers doesn't offer genetically enhanced long-distance runners a proper challenge, then they'll run it only as part of a much longer distance— perhaps as part of a posthuman marathon of 421.95 kilometers.

McKibben imagines genetically enhanced marathoners winning without having to try hard. Winning will require nothing more than the correct operation of competitors' internal accelerators. I find this unlikely. In biological terms, trying hard is essentially the allocation of additional resources toward an activity deemed especially important. This is what human marathoners are doing when they put everything they have into sprinting over the final 100 meters. Cars can't try hard. They have no capacity to decide to transfer resources normally required for functions such as maintenance of the air conditioning system or the operation of the brake lights, to boosting speed. Posthuman marathoners who are, like cars, incapable of trying hard will probably lose to those who are capable of mobilizing additional resources. The winners of posthuman marathons may even try harder than the winners of human marathons. That is, they may have an even greater capacity to channel resources normally required for other bodily or mental functions into long-distance running performances.[2]

Or course, these superhuman levels of effort may be possible only because of prenatal genetic modifications. But posthuman marathoners can acknowledge this fact even as they take pleasure in and accept credit for their achievements. Their attitude needn't be all that dissimilar to that of a God-fearing gold medalist who can acknowledge a debt to the creator while also taking pride in victory. In both cases, competitors have turned what they were born with into exceptional performances.

Vicariously Participating in Exceptional Performances

So, being "plain boring" cannot be the problem with performance enhancers. Nonetheless, enhancers may disengage us from sport in an important way. The question here is what the achievements of posthuman marathoners will mean to human spectators. Our interest in sport is governed by a species of *local value*. A locally valuable thing draws part of its worth from its relationship with those who value it. Paradigm cases are attachments to family, friends, and perhaps to nations, and these have received intensive philosophical scrutiny.[3] Although certain varieties of local values, the valuing of family and friends, for example, are high on the list of those that contribute meaning to our lives, there is some controversy about their relationship to the universal values prescribed by many moral theories.[4]

Local values shouldn't just be asserted. They require plausible rationales. The local value that corresponds to our interest in identifying directs us to take an interest in the sporting successes and failures of beings relevantly like us. Unenhanced human spectators are drawn to the achievements of unenhanced human competitors because we recognize them as pushing up against the limits of our own activities. Their exceptional performances tell us something about what we could achieve, or might have achieved had we been more fortunate, dedicated, and talented. We share many of the competitors' limitations, and this commonality gives us a unique access to and interest in their exceptional achievements.

Differently empowered beings would lack both this distinctive first-person access to and enjoyment of exceptional human performances. They would be, as a consequence, unlikely to care about how close to two hours human marathoners are capable of running. We would have a correspondingly diminished interest in their achievements. Aliens and posthumans may engage in sporting competitions that are exciting to them, challenges that engage their particular local values. But these competitions would not have the same allure for an audience of unenhanced human beings, even if we recognize that they are objectively exceptional. We would rather watch Usain Bolt run 100 meters in 9.58 seconds than see athletically superior posthumans or aliens run that distance much more quickly.

The terminology of a prominent theory of the human mind offers a convenient way to describe the nature of the perspective of unfit, unmotivated human beings on the achievements of elite athletes and the enjoyment we get out of viewing them.[5] Simulation theory addresses the problem of how we predict and explain how other human beings behave.[6] It holds that we represent the mental processes that cause the behavior of other humans by simulating those processes in our minds. The results enable us to predict what they will do, and to explain why they did what they did. For example, we see a hungry person poised before a large bowl of spaghetti bolognaise. We imagine ourselves hungry in that circumstance. The output of our simulation is likely to be a desire to eat. Simulation theory's great advantage is that it solves the problem of how we predict and explain the behavior of other human beings without requiring us to know a massive collection of facts about them. We use our own psychological processes to simulate theirs. We take this mental machinery "offline" so that it produces predictions and explanations of others rather than causing us to act in certain ways. When we simulate the mental processes of the hungry person, we understand that *she* desires to eat the pasta. The output of the simulation isn't a desire that *we* eat.

Simulation theory assumes sufficient similarity between the individual doing the simulating and the individual being simulated. If the mental processes of intelligent aliens or computers are significantly different from our own, then our simulations will not be of much use in predicting or explaining their behavior.

Gregory Currie has appealed to simulation theory to explain the experience of reading fiction (for example, Currie and Ravenscroft, 2003; Currie, 1997). He claims that we simulate when we read a work of fiction. We engage emotionally with the pleasures and pains of fictional characters by simulating their mental states. "If our imagining goes well, it will tell us something about how we would respond to the situation, and what it would be like to experience it" (1997, p. 56).

Simulation theory describes well our engagement with sport. Attentive readers of Tolstoy's *Anna Karenina* vicariously experience the central character's loves and disappointments. We get something similar out of watching sport. It's occasionally useful to be able to predict the behavior of someone seated in front of a bowl of spaghetti. But doing so is not especially exciting—unless perhaps the eater is involved in a spaghetti-eating competition for the *Guinness Book of Records*. Simulating the mental processes behind great performances enables us to feel some of the exhilaration the performers experience. We identify with elite sportspeople and vicariously participate in their triumphs and disappointments. When we simulate a great soccer goal, an incredible tennis passing shot, a daring queen sacrifice in chess, or an amazing boxing combination, we sample the exhilaration that accompanies them. We watch elite sports to vicariously experience exceptional performances and to learn something about what is possible for human beings.

Consider two descriptions of the pivotal event in the 1986 FIFA World Cup soccer quarter-final match between Argentina and England.

1. Diego Maradona scored a goal in the fifty-sixth minute.
2. "Fed by Hector Enrique, Maradona turned through 180 degrees out on the right, on the halfway line, before slipping between Peter Reid and Peter Beardsley. Next he sped inside centre-back Terry Butcher and fended off a challenge from Terry Fenwick, who had been distracted by the lurking presence of the advancing Jorge Valdano. Maradona slalomed on deep into the penalty box, waited for Peter Shilton to step from his line then dummied left before stepping right to slip the ball past the keeper and over the line just as the recovering Butcher launched another, vain tackle" (*Telegraph.co.uk,* 2007).

The second description makes exciting reading because it engages our simulation machinery. It guides us through the movements Maradona performed as he worked the ball though half the England team and encourages us to imagine doing the same. We get to feel something of Maradona's exhilaration when he completes the movement. Masochists may instead choose to simulate the mental states of the English defenders.

Our identification with the participants in elite sport requires that the athletes are sufficiently similar to us in some ways, even as their prowess is sufficiently different to generate such exceptional performances. The vicarious participation enabled by simulation is possible because of some characteristics that top human performers share with the rest of us. To paraphrase the 1992 Gatorade commercial featuring basketball legend Michael Jordan, to "be like Mike," Mike has to be sufficiently like us.

Anyone who has attempted to jog up and down their street has some insight into the experiences of Paula Radcliffe when she was producing her record-breaking performances. While Garry Kasparov may be the best human chess player there has ever been, even a thoroughly mediocre player can move the chess pieces as he and Anatoly Karpov moved them in the celebrated sixteenth game of their 1985 match. We can read Kasparov's annotations and thereby sample the pleasure he experienced in defeating the world champion.

Our interest in fiction is local in the same way as our interest in sport. There is no universal requirement that the central characters in stories be human. Indeed, it would be surprising if humans were the central characters of posthuman or alien novels. But we enjoy fictions whose central characters are human. Nonhuman characters who engage our interest are depicted with familiarly human psychologies—think of the bunny rabbits in Richard Adams's novel *Watership Down* and the hobbits in J. R. R. Tolkien's *Lord of the Rings*. If we choose to become posthuman, then our tastes in fiction and sport will change. But we aren't posthuman yet.

Chess-playing Computers and Robot Pitchers

The performances of Maradona and Kasparov are interesting because we recognize them as exceptional. Performance-enhancing drugs and modifications promise sporting exploits that will be even more exceptional. So why shouldn't we find such enhanced performances even more interesting?

Leon Kass and Eric Cohen address the problem of chess computers that appear to play chess even better than the best human players. They insist that chess will continue to be a game in which one human plays another in an era of apparent computer supremacy over the chess board because "only we can play chess, that is, as human beings, as genuine chess players." Computers do nothing more than "play" chess. That is why no one would "watch a 'match' between two chess-playing computers." It's also the reason no one would watch "a baseball game that pitted robot pitchers against automatic batting machines" (2008, p. 38).

We should be suspicious of arguments that restrict chess (or baseball) to human beings. Bonobos taught the rules of chess should lose the majority of the games they play because they're not very good players, not due to disqualification on the grounds of species-membership. Computers moving chess pieces around the board in ways that deliberately conform with the rules of the game with the aim of checkmating an opponent are playing chess, not merely "playing" it. The key difference between Deep Blue and the bonobo player is simply that the computer is better, sufficiently so to beat the best humans.

Kass and Cohen credit the designers of chess programs with the desire to build something able to "'play' perfect chess." This, they suggest, is not what human chess players are trying to do. Kasparov would, doubtless, love to play perfect chess. But his goal in preparing for his 1985 match against then-world champion Anatoly Karpov was simply to win. The IBM programmers of the chess computer Deep Blue had a similar goal when preparing their charge for the 1997 match against Kasparov. They wanted to win. Perfect chess, whatever that is, would have been a wonderful achievement, but all they really needed was for Deep Blue to play better than Kasparov.

But Kass and Cohen are right to say that we will maintain our interest in human players even after chess programs routinely beat us. This shouldn't be too surprising. We watch human 1,500-meter runners even though we know that any used car lot contains machines that beat them with ease. Kass and Cohen observe that "the computer 'plays' the game rather differently—with no uncertainty, no nervousness, no sweaty palms, no active mind, and, most crucially, with no desires or hopes regarding future success." Their point survives removing the scare quotes around "plays." Our simulations include the fear that our opponent might have spotted a flaw in our cunning plan, and joy when it/he/she makes the moves that we predicted. We enjoy watching the games of individuals who genuinely feel these things. Chess-players who do not have these experiences are not particularly interesting objects of imaginative identification (see Krauthammer, 1996).

The absence of keenly felt experiences is not the only obstacle to the pleasurable simulation of chess-playing computers. Computers approach the game differently from the way we do. According to its IBM programmers, Deep Blue's chess brain contained a database with about 700,000 games. It could generate positions and evaluate them using a function integrating four distinct measures of chess success at a speed of 200 million positions per second.[7] Contrary to the opinion of Kass and Cohen, this is one way to play chess. We could attempt to play this way. Deep Blue's programmers almost certainly tested its algorithms in their heads, playing though short sequences of moves, as a first check of their viability. A human who attempted to implement Deep Blue's algorithms, reducing the computer's rate of generating and evaluating positions from 200 million per second to around one position every five minutes, and the size of its database from 700,000 to a small number of partially remembered games, might find himself having to explain how he managed to lose to a chess-playing bonobo.

Our simulation machinery can help us with Deep Blue's chess play. We can, to some extent, get into the head of a cheetah as it races to bring down a gazelle. It can be exciting to vicariously experience the activities of beings very unlike us. But this psychological tourism differs from the motivation that draws us to sport. Those who watch sport are striving to simulate performances. Our sporting heroes become, for the duration of their performances at least, our role models. Their exceptional achievements can tell us something about our own limits.

In these scenarios, our interest in identifying is directed specifically at sporting performances and the capacities that generate them, not necessarily about the performer's character. Those who love the operas of Richard Wagner sometimes point out that their enjoyment of *Tristan and Isolde* does not imply an endorsement of Wagner the man. There's an analogous point about our imaginative identification with elite athletes. After quitting soccer, Maradona was newsworthy principally for his serial philandering and cocaine abuse. You may find these behaviors collectively more morally reprehensible than cheating in sport. When told about them, your view about Maradona, the man, could change accordingly. But marital infidelity and drug abuse, especially after one's retirement from elite sport, are not the barriers to identifying with sporting achievements that performance-enhancing drugs are. When we watch sport we don't attempt to simulate a competitor's psychology in its entirety—something we may not want to do in Maradona's case. We simulate only those aspects of their psychologies directly relevant to the performance. Performance-enhancing drugs are either an obstacle to this imaginative act or make it less enjoyable.

The Interest in Identifying versus the Interest in Extremes

Our interest in identifying places limits on how good the performances of elite athletes should be. Performances should be sufficiently good that we enjoy simulating them, but they should not be so good that they are well beyond what beings like us can do. In this case we simulate them only with great difficulty and get less out of doing so. Their performances are less likely to tell us something about what we might achieve, or might have achieved.

Simulation doesn't generate our only interest in sport. Consider the confession of David Owen, a *Financial Times* journalist, about his experience as a spectator of the single most famous instance of drug cheating: "I have a guilty secret. I think Ben Johnson's 'victory' in the men's 100m at the 1988 Seoul Olympics is just about the most exciting 10 seconds of sport I have ever witnessed" (2006). If the number of clips of Ben Johnson's race available on Youtube is any indication, then Owen may not be Johnson's only secret admirer.

The excitement that Johnson's performance elicits appeals to a different interest in sport, an interest in extremes. The people of Victorian England were spurred by this interest to attend exhibitions of the world's tallest, shortest, strongest, and hairiest humans. Johnson's 9.84 second fascinates because it was, at that time, a behavioral extreme—the fastest 100-meter dash in history. Humans are not the only things that engage our interest in extremes. It explains the popularity of Discovery Channel documentaries on the biggest dinosaurs and highest mountains.

The interest in extremes is a relatively insignificant contributor to our over-all enjoyment of sport. It does not explain the durability of our commitment. For example, how often do you pay to see an exhibition featuring the world's tallest human? You may go once to satisfy your curiosity, but I suspect you're unlikely to go more often than that. Once you've been into the tent with the world's tallest human being, how likely are you to pay the dollar to enter the tent with the world's second tallest human being? Sports fans, by contrast, tune in and turn up on a weekly, or even daily, basis. This week's sporting per-formance can give pleasure by engaging our simulation machinery even if we know that it is objectively less impressive than last week's. People who remem-ber Maradona's goal of the century still derive immense enjoyment from soccer games that do not produce goals of nearly that quality. They don't watch cover-age of the match of the week in the expectation that it will contain goals that surpass Maradona's.

WADA's Position on Synthetic EPO

Our interest in identifying offers a rationale for regulating elite sports. We prefer to watch performances that are both exceptional and produced by athletes who are relevantly similar to us. This rationale supports the measures taken by WADA. Consider, in particular, the current ban on synthetic EPO.

One important influence on success in endurance sports is a competitor's sup-ply of oxygen-carrying hemoglobin. Competitors whose blood contains a higher percentage of hemoglobin cycle up hills more quickly and are less likely to burn out before marathon finish line. The hematocrit (HCT) is a measure of the pro-portion of blood volume that is occupied by red blood cells, transporters of he-moglobin. In adult men, HCTs mostly range from 41 to 50 percent. The normal value for adult women is between 36 and 44 percent.

One way in which a competitor can increase his or her HCT is by injecting a synthetic version of erythropoietin (EPO), a hormone produced by the kidney that regulates the production of red blood cells. According to one estimate, elite cyclists boost their performance by 5 percent for every 10 percent increase in the volume of their red blood cells (Shermer, 2008). In elite sports, 5 percent can be the difference between first and nowhere. Some competitors using synthetic EPO have boosted their hematocrits to 60 percent and beyond.

There is a significant downside to using synthetic EPO to increase red blood cell count. Boosting HCT significantly increases the risk of stroke or heart attack.

It is this combination of enhancement of sporting performances and endangerment of health that places synthetic EPO among substances banned by WADA.[8]

Is WADA Inconsistent?

The philosopher Julian Savulescu has accused WADA of inconsistency (Savulescu, Foddy, and Clayton, 2004; Savulescu and Foddy, 2007). He makes the point that WADA permits athletes to supplement training's propensity to boost hematocrits through other measures. One of these is altitude training. People who live at high altitudes tend to have higher volumes of hemoglobin to cope with the thinner atmosphere. Lowlanders who train at high altitude before a major event can sufficiently boost their hematocrits to gain a competitive advantage. One can save on travel expenses and use a hypoxic air machine to reduce the concentration of oxygen in the air breathed during a workout. Or one can achieve a higher HCT by being the beneficiary of an accident of birth. The Finnish endurance skier Eero Mäntyranta is an example of a competitor who possessed high levels of hemoglobin by luck. A rare genetic mutation meant that he had between 40 and 50 percent more hemoglobin than other competitors. Initially suspected of cheating, he was cleared when the source of his advantage was found to be natural.

According to Savulescu, "There is no difference between elevating your blood count by altitude training, by using a hypoxic air machine, or by taking EPO. But the last is illegal. Some competitors have high HCTs and an advantage by luck. Some can afford hypoxic air machines" (Savulescu, Foddy, and Clayton, 2004, p. 668). What of risks to health? These exist whether a competitor has achieved the performance-enhancing level by training at altitude, by using a hypoxic air machine, as a result of an accident of birth, or by injecting synthetic EPO. It is the end result—higher than normal blood hemoglobin—that both confers the competitive advantage and imperils health. Savulescu proposes that we should ban performance enhancers only when they exceed a threshold of risk to athletes' health. Performance enhancers do not have to be entirely risk free to be allowed. We expect elite athletes to push their bodies to their limits. Cars driven to their limits risk mechanical failure, and so do human bodies. Savulescu argues that we should not exclude performance enhancers that bring risks commensurate with those ordinarily part of elite sport. Whether a competitor is sufficiently at risk of stroke or heart attack to be banned from competition is something that doctors and not WADA bureaucrats can best decide.

The consistency argument challenges us to find a moral difference between injecting EPO and using any of the techniques permitted by WADA to increase the oxygen-carrying capacity of blood. Even if it cannot meet Savulescu's challenge and find a moral difference between synthetic EPO and the various other ways of boosting competitors' hematocrits, WADA is correct to ban synthetic EPO for at least three reasons.

1. No competitor has an antecedent interest in injecting synthetic EPO to gain a competitive advantage. Attempts to prohibit other ways to boost hematocrits do, in contrast, infringe legitimate antecedent interests.
2. A rule permitting synthetic EPO is open-ended in a way that conflicts with our interest in identifying.
3. A rule banning synthetic EPO is more practical than a rule banning other techniques for boosting hematocrits.

No One Has an Antecedent Interest in Using Synthetic EPO to Gain a Competitive Advantage

There is much that is arbitrary about the rules of sport. Sprinters run 100 meters and not 95 meters or 105 meters simply because meters are a convenient unit of measure and 100 is a round number. The competitor who was ahead of the eventual gold medallist in all but the final meters of the Olympic sprint final may make the point that he would have won had the race been over at 95 meters. But he cannot claim that he came to the race with an antecedent interest in the race's being slightly shorter. Antecedent interests are independent of the rules of a sport.

The most obvious way you might have an antecedent interest in a certain method of boosting your hematocrit is by being born with a genome that elevates your hemoglobin. Eero Mäntyranta was born with a rare mutation in the gene that regulates the body's production of EPO. It would be unjust to exclude him just because we happen to know more about the precise mechanism of his inborn advantage than we do about the inborn advantages that Tiger Woods brings to golf or Roger Federer brings to tennis.

There is a difference between banning Eero Mäntyranta and banning a technique for modifying competitors' DNA to be like Mäntyranta's. Mäntyranta's claim on competing as he was born differs from the claim another competitor might make on modifying his or her DNA to be like Mäntyranta's. The processes that formed Mäntyranta's genome acted independently of the rules of Olympic competition. The act of genetically modifying yourself or others so as to maximize the chances of winning gold medals in Olympic events is, in contrast, not independent of competitions; its purpose is competitive advantage.

Some competitors might claim an antecedent interest in a genetic modification that boosts levels of hemoglobin. For example, some people are seriously anemic. Synthetic EPO is one treatment for this condition, but we can imagine a more permanent genetic fix. Injecting EPO to treat serious anemia or modifying genomes to prevent forms of anemia that have a genetic cause are independent of the rules of competition and should therefore not be excluded. A principle distinguishing between modifications that are independent of the rules of competition and those that are not is easily stated. Problems arise in its implementation. Consider the debate surrounding South African sprinter Oscar Pistorius.[9] Pistorius was born with a congenital malformation of his legs. He had an antecedent interest in mobility, to be able not only to walk but also to run, activities that most of us take for granted. To what degree the design of his Cheetah Flex-Foot carbon-fiber transtibial artificial limbs was to promote his antecedent interest and to what degree it was to gain athletic advantage in Olympic sprint events remains a question.

Another way in which competitors may have an antecedent interest in a certain means of boosting performance is for that means to be cultural property. Taken in an appropriate way, coffee can be strongly performance enhancing. A ban on coffee would be a ban on a beverage that many competitors consider an essential part of their daily routines. Drug-taking may have been routine among East German Olympians. But this does not make anabolic steroids or any other banned substance cultural property. The interest of East German coaches in anabolic steroids clearly postdated the making of the rules of the sports they used it to gain advantage in. People tend not to conceal their culture's traditional practices. Herein lies the difference between Italians' traditional espresso and the administration of anabolic steroids by East German coaches. The former is openly embraced as cultural property. The latter was not.

The cultural property argument enables a partial response to Savulescu's consistency argument. An entitlement to object X as cultural property is not also an entitlement to any other object that resembles X in its propensity to enhance performance. Suppose recombinant DNA technology provides a compound that once injected has an effect on performance identical that of a strong espresso coffee. The fact that competitors can claim coffee as cultural property does not also mean that they can lay claim to the recombinant DNA product.

A ban on training at altitude would also conflict with an antecedent interest that some competitors have in living in certain parts of the world. If you live in the Andes, then you have an antecedent interest in continuing to live there. Requiring you to move to sea level to become eligible for elite competition would violate this interest.

A Rule Permitting Synthetic EPO Is Open-ended in a Way That Conflicts with Our Interest in Identifying

A further justification for a ban on certain drugs and modifications is that they have open-ended consequences for the performances of elite athletes. This open-endedness poses a threat to spectators' identification with their sporting heroes.

The natural secretion of EPO by the kidneys sets limits on the quantity of hemoglobin that altitude training or hypoxic air machines can produce. The ability of these practices to enhance performance and their threat to our capacity to imaginatively identify is therefore limited. Synthetic EPO, in contrast, avoids internal regulatory limits by bypassing the kidneys. It is injected directly into competitors' bloodstreams, enabling them to achieve hematocrits of 60 percent and beyond.

Savulescu's suggestion that we should ban drugs and modifications that unduly threaten competitors' health and well-being offers only a partial response to this point. The act of boosting an athlete's hematocrit to 60 percent significantly increases the risk of heart attack and stroke as it undermines the spectator interest in identifying. It is convenient that performances that are accessible to us tend to be safe.

However, consider how athletes could soon be boosting their reserves of oxygen. Robert A. Freitas Jr. has described something called a respirocyte, a one-micron-wide nanobot designed as a replacement for hemoglobin. It is currently a merely theoretical entity. But should Freitas's dreams be realized, respirocytes could be introduced into human bodies, dramatically outperforming hemoglobin in keeping our tissues oxygenated. Respirocytes could carry 236 times the quantity of oxygen as the hemoglobin they replace. This means that a few cubic centimeters of them could "exactly replace the gas carrying capacity of the patient's entire 5.4 liters of blood." Respirocytes could "enable a healthy person to sprint at top speed for at least 15 minutes without breathing, or to sit underwater at the bottom of a swimming pool for hours" (Frietas, 2002).[10]

Perhaps Freitas is right—replacing our cumbersome, inefficient hemoglobin is the best thing that we could do for ourselves. When we have done this, we will acquire an interest in the exceptional performances of athletes who have them. We'll have comparatively little interest in the successes and failures of competitors with biological hemoglobin. Until this time, we should exclude them from the elite sports that we watch, buy tickets for, and otherwise subsidize.

When they are first declared safe for human use, respirocytes and the technologies that substitute them for hemoglobin are likely to be expensive and available only to the very rich. Respirocytes should be banned from elite sport if they are restricted to billionaires—unless, that is, we want to be treated to the unedifying spectacle of Donald Trump, his arteries coursing with respirocytes, beating Haile Gebrselassie in the Olympic marathon. We should change the rules of sport only when respirocytes are widely available and popular among spectators of sport.

Banning Synthetic EPO Is More Practical Than Banning Other Techniques for Boosting Hematocrits

The reason we are right to ban synthetic EPO is simply that it can be banned. The practicality of banning performance enhancers should not be conflated with whether or not the ban can be successfully enforced. EPO cheats are difficult to detect. Ten years elapsed from the addition of synthetic EPO to WADA's list of banned substances until the organization felt that it could administer a sufficiently reliable test. Those who test positive routinely challenge the results. But just because cheats are difficult to detect does not mean we should not attempt to detect them. It is worth pursuing corporate fraudsters even if when we know that many of them are too clever and well resourced to be caught.

Another point about the practicality of banning synthetic EPO relates to the distinction between legal and illegal ways of boosting the oxygen-carrying capacity of blood. Today, those who give synthetic EPO to competitors know that they are breaking the rules. Trainers and competitors recognize the practice as out of the ordinary, different from the things they typically do to prepare for competition.

EPO must be injected. On seeing a strange syringe, few people immediately think that they should inject its contents. We must normally be given pretty persuasive reasons either to inject a substance or to allow it to be injected into us.

Similar points apply to performance enhancers that are ingested. We are usually careful to establish that what we are put into our mouths falls into the category of food. Herein lies a difference between coffee and some stimulants that come in tablet form. We recognize coffee as food, but not tablets. This makes a rule permitting the former but banning the latter possible to comply with.

There are also practical difficulties for Savulescu's standard. His determination to ban competitors whose hematocrits exceed a certain level does not translate directly into a rule telling them how much EPO they can inject. Competitors with naturally low percentages of hemoglobin would presumably be allowed to inject more than Eero Mäntyranta, for example. This places competitors in a difficult situation. Under Savulescu's proposed regime, they will want to inject sufficient EPO to get as close as they can to the therapeutic maximum without overdosing. Many are likely to exceed this maximum in their attempts. There is also the factor that medical opinions about the effects on health have a tendency to change over time. Competitors may find that the latest issue of the *Lancet* has changed the received medical view on how much synthetic EPO is safe.

A ban on altitude training is likely to be much more difficult to implement than a ban on synthetic EPO. Presumably there would be a quota of training at altitude that a competitor would not be allowed to exceed. Some competitive cyclists live at elevated altitude. They would have to relocate to ensure that a sufficient percentage of their training is done at an acceptable altitude. We can imagine the World Anti-Altitude-training Agency (WAAA) fitting competitors with tracking beacons to determine if legal quotas are being exceeded. This regulatory regime is likely to see cyclists returning from what would seem to them to be perfectly ordinary training rides up and down the hills of their town to learn that they have inadvertently exceeded their allowable monthly quota of training at altitude.

A ban on hypoxic air machines might be more easily implemented. The most congenial view of Tour de France cyclists is that their training is a condensed and exaggerated version of what ordinary weekend cyclists do. Hypoxic air machines certainly are not part of this image of sport. But a ban on the machines would, nonetheless, be quite difficult to implement. It involves restricting the kinds of places that competitors can train. We expect elite athletes to train at extremely well-equipped gymnasiums. A hypoxic air machine is an unusual piece of gym equipment, to be sure. It would be easier to ban hypoxic air machines than it would be to ban training at altitude. But a ban on injections of EPO is considerably easier to implement than a ban on either of these practices.

Why Elite Athletes Need New Self-conceptions

It is one thing to assert that drug cheating is wrong. Actually doing something about it seems difficult in an era in which there are larger and larger rewards for victory and biotechnologists keep finding ways to enhance performance that are ever more powerful and difficult to detect.

I doubt we will ever eliminate cheating entirely. There will be cheating in any domain of activity that rewards excellence. But there is some chance we can reduce cheating to a level at which it is no longer discussed as a threat to the very existence of elite sport. We need to change the way elite athletes conceive of themselves so that they are more in line with the expectations of their spectators.

Ben Johnson's statements following his disgrace provide ample evidence that elite sportspeople's self-conceptions are disconnected from spectators' view of them. The public tends to place him together with Tonya Harding and Mike Tyson, in a category of individuals known for things that happened in a sporting context but which were not properly part of sport. But this isn't how Johnson thinks of himself. On one of the many occasions that he was questioned about his treatment after the 1988 Olympics, Johnson said, "Don't tell me I cheated the system because that's [expletive]. I didn't get treated fairly by the system. They cast me out and they were jealous because I turned in the fastest time ever run by a human and it was impossible at the time" (Grossfeld, 2005).

The quest for victory seems essential to elite sports. Johnson can justifiably say that he was doing all he could to run fast. He was doing all he could to satisfy the audience interest in extremes. But Johnson was wrong to think that our principal interest is in how fast he runs. Our interest in exceptional performance is tempered with a desire that elite performances be relevant to us. We enjoy simulating performances at the limits of human capacity. Performances produced with the help of Stanozolol are less apt for simulation. We get more enjoyment out of watching a clean athlete run slower.

In the years since the Seoul Olympics, Johnson sometimes has seemed like an actor who protests his dumping from the lead role in a production of *Hamlet*. Even if he perfectly remembered all of Hamlet's 1,495 lines, missed none of his entrances, and was excellent in the fight scenes, it isn't worth much if the actor failed to convey Hamlet's humanity to his audience. No one is in doubt that there are ways human beings could be modified that could lead them to traverse 100 meters incredibly quickly. The remarkable thing was that an unmodified human being could do it. This was how Johnson was fraudulently presenting himself.

ACKNOWLEDGMENTS

This chapter has benefited from comments from Gregory Kaebnick, Simon Keller, and an audience in the Philosophy Program at Victoria University of Wellington.

NOTES

1. See, for example, the comments of Leon Kass and Eric Cohen that "playing to the crowd and satisfying its tastes is at bottom a deformation of athletics, an adulteration imported from the theatre" (2008, p. 40).

2. For an interesting discussion of the South African amputee sprinter, Oscar Pistorius, see Gregory Kaebnick (2007). Kaebnick points out that concerns over whether Pistorius is enhanced are independent of the issue of the remarkable nature of his performances.

3. For a recent treatment, see Keller (2007).

4. A widely cited paper that addresses the apparent tension between consequentialist moral theory and friendship is Railton (1988).

5. Simulation theory affords a particularly intuitive presentation of our interest in identifying. But the account of our enjoyment of sport can be made independently of simulation theory. We learn something about the achievement of elite performers, or identify with them, by reflecting on some of our own psychological states and dispositions.

6. For a useful introduction to simulation theory, see Gordon (2009).

7. See www.research.ibm.com/deepblue/meet/html/d.3.2.html.

8. See the World Anti-Doping Code 2009, section 4.3. The code is available at www.wada-ama.org/en/World-Anti-Doping-Program/Sports-and-Anti-Doping-Organizations/The-Code/.

9. Kaebnick (2007) concludes that Pistorius can legitimately be excluded from Olympic competition.

10. For more on the respirocyte, see www.foresight.org/nanomedicine/gallery/Species/Respirocytes.html.

REFERENCES

Currie, G. 1997. "The Moral Psychology of Fiction." In *Art and Its Messages: Meaning, Morality, and Society,* ed. S. Davies, pp. 49–58. University Park: Pennsylvania State University Press.

Currie, G., and I. Ravenscroft. 2003. *Recreative Minds: Imagination in Philosophy and Psychology.* New York: Oxford University Press.

Freitas, R. 2002. "Robots in the Bloodstream: The Promise of Nanomedicine." *KurzweilAI.net,* February 26. www.kurzweilai.net/robots-in-the-bloodstream-the-promise-of-nanomedicine.

Gordon, R. 2009. "Folk Psychology as Mental Simulation." *Stanford Encyclopedia of Philosophy.* http://plato.stanford.edu/entries/folkpsych-simulation/.

Grossfeld, S. 2005. "Johnson Has Been Slow to Admit Wrongdoing." *Boston Globe,* April 28.

Kaebnick, G. 2007. "Human Nature and the Nature of Sports." *Bioethics Forum,* June 18. www.bioethicsforum.org/Oscar-Pistorius-human-nature-sports.asp.

Kass, L., and E. Cohen. 2008. "For the Love of the Game." *New Republic* 238 (5): 34–42.

Keller, S. 2007. *The Limits of Loyalty.* Cambridge, U.K.: Cambridge University Press.

Krauthammer, C. 1996. "Deep Blue Funk." *Time,* February 26.

McKibben, B. 2003. *Enough: Staying Human in an Engineered Age.* New York: Times Books.

Owen, D. 2006. "Chemically Enhanced." *Financial Times,* February 11.

Railton, P. 1988. "Alienation, Consequentialism, and the Demands of Morality." In *Consequentialism and Its Critics,* ed. S. Scheffler, pp. 93–133. Oxford: Oxford University Press.

Savulescu, J., and B. Foddy. 2007. "Ethics of Performance Enhancement in Sport: Drugs and Gene Doping." In *Principles of Health Care Ethics,* 2nd ed., ed. R. E. Ashcroft, A. Dawson, H. Draper, and J. R. McMillan, pp. 511–20. London: John Wiley & Sons.

Savulescu, J., B. Foddy, and M. Clayton. 2004. "Why We Should Allow Performance Enhancing Drugs in Sport." *British Journal of Sports Medicine* 38:666–70.

Shermer, M. 2008. "The Doping Dilemma." *Scientific American,* March.

Telegraph.co.uk. 2007. "The Greatest Goals of All Time." July 4. www.telegraph.co.uk/sport/main.jhtml?xml=/sport/2007/07/16/nosplit/urgreatestgoals.xml.

CHAPTER ELEVEN

Commonsense Morality and the Idea of Nature

What We Can Learn from Thinking about "Therapy"

William A. Galston, Ph.D.

Our challenge is to understand whether the appeal to nature helps orient judgments and practice in areas such as medicine, biotechnology, and the environment. My point of departure is a distinction between two conceptions of nature. The first is of nature as a whole, as a realm distinguished from others of equal generality. In this spirit, the Greeks distinguished between nature and convention; Kantians, between nature and freedom; modern scientists, between nature and nurture; and so on. The second conception is finer grained, nature as the "nature of"—the defining characteristics of—particular entities or species.

The conceptual architecture of language—including our normative language—reflects the "nature of" humans as a particular kind of embodied species: rational and passionate, selfish and other-directed, individuated and social, vulnerable and mortal. That is why Kant's quest for morality binding on "all rational beings as such" is doomed to failure.

The concept of health is an example of embodied normative discourse. We can understand it approximately, in rough and ready terms, as the appropriate functioning of the human body and mind. If we were different kinds of beings, our understanding of appropriate functioning would shift accordingly. We cannot rule out the possibility that our species will evolve in ways that alter the content of this concept. But this possibility reinforces the point; our operative conception of health is relative to what we are as a species.

While distinctions at this level of abstraction can be illuminating, they are unlikely to help us make progress toward resolving practical disputes. To get farther, we must employ a method I call commonsense morality.[1] We should focus on examples rather than concepts and definitions. We should move, as Aristotle recommends, from the more known to the less known. We should start with easy cases to establish what John Rawls calls "provisional fixed points"—presumptive judgments—for moral reflection. We should move from these moral particulars to concepts and principles—from the "what" to the "why"—and use them as tests that larger moral hypotheses should meet. While searching for bright-line concepts and principles, we should be satisfied, if necessary, with fuzzier demarcations and family resemblances. And we should acknowledge that the maximal closure that philosophical reflection can achieve is likely to leave an area of permanent indeterminacy that fails to resolve hard cases.

Beyond the Therapy/Enhancement Distinction?

We can approach the relation between health and nature as "nature of" through the controversy, sparked by developments in pharmacology and genetics, over the distinction between therapy and enhancement. Roughly speaking, therapy is designed to attain or restore normal functioning; enhancement is designed to go beyond the bounds of normal functioning. The President's Council on Bioethics (2003, p. 13n) argues, "The notion of 'beyond therapy' does not seem to us to define the royal road to understanding. For this, one must adopt an outlook not only 'beyond therapy' but also 'beyond the distinction between therapy and enhancement.' One needs to see the topic less in relation to medicine and its purposes, and more in relation to human beings and their purposes."

This claim is exposed to an obvious objection: the purposes of therapy—health and normal functioning—*are* human purposes. So the issue is better posed as the place of these goods within the overall moral economy of human life. Yes, terms such as "health" and "normality" are contestable, and sometimes contested. But despite a blurred periphery, they are comparatively unproblematic and retain a commonsense core that offers moral and practical guidance. Besides, it is hard to believe that moving from the therapy/enhancement distinction to a broader discussion of human purposes will narrow the zone of contestation. Rather, deep differences over the sources of meaning, purpose, and value will come to the fore.

As Thomas Murray and Eric Juengst have argued, the therapy/enhancement distinction delimits a moral boundary between domains that are guided by different kinds of considerations (Murray, 2007; Juengst, 1998). In keeping with the Aristotelian procedure I am recommending, we should begin within the four corners of the narrower debate, seeking as much clarity and agreement as the subject permits, before moving to more contested terrain.

Murray considers four difficulties with the distinction. The first difficulty is that all therapy can be understood as enhancement. In a sense, yes, he replies, but not all enhancement can be understood as therapy. The crucial point is the end in view, health and normal functioning versus some other good. He offers a similar response to the second purported difficulty, that some biomedical interventions aim unequivocally at health but are clearly a form of enhancement. (For example, vaccines work by enhancing the immune system's capacity to respond to an infectious agent.) As he notes, vaccines are "clearly directed at the usual aims of therapy: preserving health and preventing disease" (p. 495).

The third objection raises more complex questions. For some interventions, such as human growth hormone (HGH), there is a continuum of applications stretching from therapy to enhancement, and it by no means clear where to draw the line. While this is a genuine problem in practice, it is not confined to the therapy/enhancement distinction. Most concepts have a solid core and fuzzy perimeter, and the latter does not negate the former. There are clear instances, even when we cannot agree on how to characterize hard cases. (I shall return to this point later.)

Murray considers a final difficulty: the same goal may be reached by a variety of means, only some of which are biomedical. While this is no doubt true, it is not clear how it calls the therapy/enhancement distinction into question. If depression can be relieved by SSRIs but also by talk therapy, meditation and prayer, or even exercise, there may be good arguments to begin with other means before turning to SSRIs. Nevertheless, the drugs remain therapeutic—that is, directed toward normal and healthy functioning.

Whatever other work it may do, the therapy/enhancement distinction does not draw a line between what is permitted and forbidden. It is not the case that all enhancements are morally wrong, or even questionable. Conversely, the fact that X would promote Y's health and normal functioning is a presumptive but not dispositive reason to do X. Rather, the distinction points to a structure of justification. The purpose of therapy is to restore health or ensure normal development and functioning. Enhancement serves other purposes whose validity and importance must be assessed. And the distinction often demarcates an ethical boundary between the presumptively obligatory and the optional. If an individual is experiencing a life-threatening breathing obstruction, any competent physician in the area has a prima facie obligation to render assistance; not so for someone who wants cosmetic surgery to improve the appearance of his abdomen or her nose.

Commonsense Morality and the Therapy/Enhancement Distinction

What follows is a series of examples designed to illustrate both that solid core and the fuzzy perimeter of the therapy/enhancement distinction.

The Normal Healthy Baby

Consider the desire of virtually all parents-to-be for a "normal, healthy baby." They have in mind the following: (1) normal form, including the right number of limbs in the appropriate places and the absence of significant deformities; (2) normal organ function; and (3) the capacity for normal development. To the extent that infants fall short along one or more of these dimensions, we commonly say that they have birth "defects," a term that would have no meaning absent some rough-and-ready concept of a nondefective condition. Similarly, I have yet to hear of an HIV-positive pregnant woman who wants her baby to be born with that condition. There are clear cases of disease, and we have no doubt that they are conditions to be avoided or cured if possible.

Activities of the World Health Organization

Similar considerations apply to groups such as the World Health Organization. We do not typically spend a great deal of time arguing about the normative valence of malaria or polio or river blindness. They are human bads, and the point is to resist and, if possible, eradicate them from the face of the earth. (Recall the global jubilation when smallpox was expunged from the human species and confined to laboratories.) To be sure, we can and do argue about the allocation of scarce resources among efforts to fight bad conditions. Often our judgments are shaped by contestable assessments of the social impact of different diseases or by the bang we can get for a limited number of bucks. But we are not arguing about whether these diseases are bad. Our moral vocabulary presupposes that they are.

Therapy up to a Point, Enhancement beyond It

I turn now to cases that illustrate how therapy and enhancement can be related as points on a continuum. Consider, first, the not-entirely-fictitious case of a world-class cyclist afflicted with testicular cancer. Both surgical and hormonal treatments can have the effect of reducing the body's production of testosterone. It seems uncontroversial that treatments designed to restore the level of testosterone the cyclist enjoyed before the onset of the disease would count as therapy. The difficulty is that treatment need not stop there. One can imagine the cyclist receiving regular injections that would elevate his testosterone level significantly above the predisease baseline—a clear case of enhancement.

When a nation's organizing committee wrestled with such a case more than a decade ago, some members wondered whether the athlete in question would take advantage of his adversity to elevate his testosterone above his predisease level. But the controversy revolved around questions of measurement and enforcement rather than conceptual or normative disagreement. As far as we know, committee members agreed in principle that simply restoring the status quo ante would be a clear case of permitted therapy rather than forbidden enhancement.

The increasingly widespread use of Ritalin poses similar issues. On the one hand, ADHD is a genuine disease with an organic basis and even genetic markers. Ritalin can regulate its symptoms in many cases, allowing children to sit still and focus normally in the classroom. In principle, this is a straightforward therapeutic intervention. On the other hand, it turns out that the drug is equally able to improve performance among individuals who do not have ADHD, and use among adults as well as children has been skyrocketing. There is a real risk that competition among parents will produce widespread use of Ritalin for enhancement as well as therapy—not to mention that both diagnosis and appropriate dosage are ambiguous in many cases (President's Council on Bioethics, 2003, pp. 74–85).

Human growth hormone (HGH) poses more complicated issues. On the one hand, most congenitally short people are capable of normal physical functioning and development. On the other hand, there is a point beyond which below-normal height impairs normal social functioning—for example, by making it harder to qualify for certain jobs and even to find marriage partners. In such circumstances, I suggest, the use of HGH to narrow the gap between these individuals and the social perimeter of normality constitutes therapy rather than enhancement.

What might this principle mean in practice? Can we make it tolerably precise and operational? Consider a personal example. I am about four inches shorter than the median American male, which probably puts me in the bottom quartile. As far as I know, I have never experienced meaningful social exclusion or disadvantage as a consequence of that fact. At the end of seventh grade I was still among the taller boys in my class. By the end of the summer, I was among the shortest, cutting short my brief career as center in pickup basketball games. Disappointing, to be sure, but hardly tragic. And even if my parents had known about my eventual height the day I was born, they would have had no reason to intervene. Indeed, they would have been wrong to do so.

But suppose they had been told that instead of five feet six inches, I would end up at three feet six inches, absent early and aggressive intervention. That is a difference of degree sufficient to constitute a difference in kind. I would have been singled out as different and subjected to ridicule. I would have experienced great difficulty finding a wife, and probably a job. If a normal social life is important for normal human development, I would have been warped to some degree. In such circumstances, the argument for therapeutic intervention becomes much stronger. For parents, it may move beyond permitted to morally obligatory.

It is a further question whether the law should regard the failure to honor such an obligation as falling within the legal definition of child neglect. Consider a related example: assume that in twenty years we know which genes are implicated in congenital deafness and how to replace them with genetic material that will ensure that infants are born able to hear. Assume that the needed resources are socially provided and that the procedure imposes minimal risks on mother and fetus. While it is not clear that making the procedure mandatory would be the right thing to do, all things considered, it is clear that important considerations point in that direction. (These considerations would bulk even larger for potential defects such as cystic fibrosis that truncate life expectancy.)

A Difficult Case: Transgender Surgery

Erik Parens invites us to reflect on individuals who experience a fundamental mismatch between their sense of themselves as male (or female) and their physical embodiment. Increasing numbers of men and women are seeking surgery to close this gap, raising the question of whether these procedures are more analogous to therapy or to enhancement.

As it happens, I know a transgendered individual—born physically male, now female—reasonably well. The decision to undergo surgery was fraught with complications and risks beyond the physical, including the possible disruption of relations with children, a parent, a partner, friends, and acquaintances. This individual certainly did not regard this transition as an optional enhancement. It stood at the farthest possible remove from cosmetic surgery. It offered, rather, a chance to repair a dysfunctional and emotionally painful defect that went to the heart of his/her life experience. At least as interpreted from the inside, the outcome was profoundly therapeutic.

The burden of proof, it seems to me, rests on those who would reject the practical force of this interpretation. This is not to say that there are no good arguments for restricting access to these surgical procedures. It is to say that at least when physicians, counselors, and patients comply with carefully crafted presurgical protocols, the reasons for proceeding outweigh the reservations that reasonable skeptics may adduce.

When Is Enhancement Justified?

I stated earlier that the distinction between therapy and enhancement does not draw a line between the permitted and the forbidden. Many forms of cosmetic surgery may appear frivolous, but it is hard to argue that they are all morally wrong, let alone that physicians should be legally debarred from performing them. Or consider the proliferating debates over enhanced performance. Where, if anywhere, should we draw the line?

As a general matter, I suggest, performance-oriented enhancements are presumptively justified when the central issue is noncompetitive performance directed toward a good separate from the action itself and where issues of individual agency in attaining that good are not central to our evaluation of the act. As the President's Council argues, there is nothing wrong with using drugs to enhance the airline pilot's alertness, to steady the neurosurgeon's hand, or to reduce a concert pianist's nervous sweat (President's Council on Bioethics, 2003, pp. 104, 292; see also Murray, 2007, p. 505). Nor would it be wrong for a sharpshooter to take performance-enhancing drugs in warfare or for a runner in a remote area under genocidal threat to take whatever may be available to enhance his speed and stamina as he races to seek assistance before it is too late.

Compare this with the much-discussed cases of competitive athletes such as Barry Bonds, Floyd Landis, and Marion Jones. There is a long list of compelling objections to what they allegedly (in Jones's and Landis's cases, admittedly) did: they broke the rules to which they had agreed to adhere, gained an unfair advantage, made use of aids not equally available to all, misrepresented what they had done, undermined the basis for comparing their performance to others (including predecessors), and claimed credit for accomplishments properly attributed to factors other than personal agency.

Yes, one may reply, but this just pushes the question back a step. Suppose that the governors of baseball, cycling, and track changed their sports fundamentally so that the use of performance-enhancing drugs was within the rules, fully public, and equally available. Then the problem would go deeper, and we would be compelled to inquire into the purposes and meanings of athletic competition.

My suggestion is that, rightly understood, this activity is intended to call forth and display the relevant excellences of human agency and that anything that weakens the connection between performance and agency contradicts the meaning and purpose of athletic competition.

To illustrate my contention, let me describe a memorable experience. I was watching golf on television on a Sunday afternoon. Tiger Woods came to the final hole tied with another player. His approach shot left him with a long, twisting downhill putt, a very difficult shot. He sized up the situation and responded with a perfect stroke; the putt curved beautifully, lost pace, and then dove into the cup. The gallery exploded; seasoned commentators were rendered mute; even the tournament's sponsor, Arnold Palmer, shook his head and smiled in rueful disbelief. All knew that they had witnessed greatness in action. Their admiration was directed toward his superb conditioning, flawless mastery of every facet of the game, iron concentration, and indomitable will. He had displayed the body, mind, and heart of a champion.

Now consider a science-fiction counterfactual. Suppose that Woods had been using specially engineered contact lenses that revealed otherwise invisible contours of the putting green and displayed the putt's length and break in graphical form. This auxiliary device would have weakened the link between the putt and his personal agency and would have changed our assessment of the deed.

Granted, the skeptic can deploy a gradation of examples designed to create a continuum between legitimate improvements in equipment and training and the story I have just told. This is where the practice of commonsense morality does real work. The existence of hard cases does not negate the moral force of clear cases. An intuitive but powerful sense of human agency is at work in our judgment of athletic competition, and despite the complexities, we know it when we see it.

The Appeal to Nature and Our Orientation in the World

Whether we are considering the physical or the spiritual dimension of human existence, the appeal to nature is at once vital and problematic. In the course of urging us to move beyond the therapy/enhancement distinction, the President's Council makes an undeniable point: the human being whose wholeness or healing is the goal of therapy is physically finite and frail. Health and normal functioning included aging and mortality. The normal eighty-five-year-old is different from the normal thirty-five-year-old. A being with the possibility of earthly immortality would not be human, at least as we now understand the term. It does not follow that it would necessarily be an error to pursue advances in medicine and biotechnology that aimed toward indefinitely prolonging human life.

Similar considerations are at work in the moral realm. Human beings have a capacity for kindness and cruelty, selfishness and altruism, justice and injustice. We may choose to evade the difficulty by resorting to a moralized or perfectionist account according to which our nature is the realization of the highest and best human possibilities. But if we begin with everyday experience, it seems far more compelling to posit the capacities for good and evil as equiprimordial.

Do these complications imply that we should set nature aside as irrelevant? I think not. As Murray puts it, "The effort to ground an ethics of enhancement on an inward-looking account of human nature fails. Not all that is natural is good, and not all unnatural enhancements are bad. But between human nature as inferior raw material and human nature as ultimate unambiguous and infallible guide to right living, there remains a third possibility: human nature as a framework for the possibilities of human flourishing. Human nature, understood as the tension between our higher longings and our worldly biology, enfolds the possibilities of such flourishing" (2007, p. 505). If Murray is right, then how we navigate that tension is morally crucial, a journey for which there is no obvious map. Parens (2005) offers one of the most compelling explorations of this terrain. The central issue, he argues, is how we should orient ourselves toward the given—that is, toward the limits of human existence. There is a continuum of possible response. At one extreme is passive resignation; at the other, Promethean hyperagency. Less extreme is the polarity of, on the one hand, gratitude for what is given and, on the other, the desire to improve on it, between the virtue of humility and the capacity for creativity.

Religions differ as to how a defensible balance is to be struck between these stances. Buddhism is usually interpreted as inclining toward gratitude and humility. By contrast, Judaism embodies a preference for activism and improvement. *Imitatio dei* means that human beings are called on to be, in the Talmudic phrase, "God's partners in creation." This implies, inter alia, a more permissive, even welcoming, attitude toward biotechnological innovation than one finds in Roman Catholicism.

This schema refines but does not resolve the question before us. One way of advancing the discussion is to recall that Aristotle, who regularly employed the idea of the ethical continuum, was never satisfied to identify what he regarded as the point of equipoise. He asked, as well, where the greatest temptation to depart from that point was located, and he recommended the practice of leaning against it. As Parens observes, the weightiest social forces today are to be found on the side of creativity rather than humility. Innovation is spurred not only by the hope of commercial gain but also by deep-seated human desires for beauty, power, and immortality. It would seem to follow that in doubtful matters the presumption should be in favor of restraint. As applied to intervening in the complex human organism, the precautionary principle points in the same direction. The rabbinic sages underscored this point; human selfishness, they noted, is the motive for producing many human goods. Even if we could excise self-interest from the human psyche in the name of moral improvement, it might be a grave mistake to do so, all things considered.

The complexities that inhere in the appeal to nature do not permit us to discard it altogether as a point of reference. Both "disease" and "disability" are privative notions denoting the absence of an important human good. Our entire moral vocabulary in this area rests on tacit assumptions about the goods of human life. If some first-year philosophy student asks why AIDS or spinal bifida is bad, what are we supposed to say? We can advert to pain or discomfort, or to impairment of some function, or to death itself, but that will not stop a sufficiently persistent student.

Ultimately, we have to say that whether through evolution or design, the broad features of the existence of our species shape certain sentiments about what is good and bad. If our species had different characteristics, our moral understanding would be different. (Imagine if we could not feel pleasure or pain, or were indifferent to the prospect of death.)

This fact helps explain some of the peculiar difficulty of moral argument concerning enhancement. If our moral vocabulary reflects some large facts about our species as it is, then we run into the moral equivalent (literally) of the difficulty

Kant explored in the *Critique of Pure Reason* regarding propositions that fall outside the framework of our empirical understanding. In this respect, among many others, I agree with Tom Murray's observation: "There is a very important distinction here between relying on the idea of the natural as the fundamental basis for an ethics of enhancement—a project unlikely to succeed—and understanding that our nature shapes the contours of our moral world. Our possibilities for flourishing are not as unfettered willful agents, but as embodied creatures whose lives and flourishing are deeply intertwined with one another" (2007, p. 514).

NOTE

1. In the rest of this paragraph, I build in part on Kaebnick (2007).

REFERENCES

Juengst, E. 1998. "What Does Enhancement Mean?" In *Enhancing Human Traits: Ethical and Social Implications,* ed. E. Parens, pp. 29–47 . Washington, D.C.: Georgetown University Press.

Kaebnick, G. E. 2007. "Putting Concerns about Nature in Context: The Case of Agricultural Biotechnology." *Perspectives in Biology and Medicine* 50, 4:572–84.

Murray, T. H. 2007. "Enhancement." In *The Oxford Handbook of Bioethics,* ed. B. Steinbock, pp. 491–515. Oxford: Oxford University Press.

Parens, E. 2005. "Authenticity and Ambivalence: Toward Understanding the Enhancement Debate." *Hastings Center Report* 35 (3): 34–41.

President's Council on Bioethics. 2003. *Beyond Therapy: Biotechnology and the Pursuit of Happiness.* Washington, D.C.

CHAPTER TWELVE

Rawls, Sports, and Liberal Legitimacy

Thomas H. Murray, Ph.D., and Peter Murray

> In addition to having these two moral powers, persons also have at any given time a determinate conception of the good that they try to achieve. Such a conception must not be understood narrowly but rather as including a conception of what is valuable in human life. Thus, a conception of the good normally consists of a more or less determinate scheme of final ends, that is, ends we want to realize for their own sake, as well as attachments to other persons and loyalties to various groups and associations. These attachments and loyalties give rise to devotions and affections, and so the flourishing of the persons and associations who are the objects of these sentiments is also part of our conception of the good. We also connect with such a conception a view of our relation to the world—religious, philosophical, and moral—by reference to which the value and significance of our ends and attachments are understood.   —JOHN RAWLS, *POLITICAL LIBERALISM*

> First: the rules of the game are in equilibrium: that is, from the start, the diamond was made just the right size, the pitcher's mound just the right distance from home plate, etc., and this makes possible the marvelous plays, such as the double play. The physical layout of the game is perfectly adjusted to the human skills it is meant to display and call into graceful exercise.
> —JOHN RAWLS, LETTER TO OWEN FISS, APRIL 18, 1981,
> ON WHY BASEBALL IS THE BEST OF ALL GAMES

> I was not successful as a ball player, as it was a game of skill.
> —CASEY STENGEL

Discussions of human nature often center on empirical questions about human tendencies and traits. Sport might be seen, then, as an expression of the natural desire for competition or domination. This way of approaching human nature makes it difficult to see how such an account could be normative, how it could help guide us in determining what we ought to do in the arena of sport. For example, it might be that human beings have an innate tendency to aggression. But this bare descriptive fact about human beings is not enough for us to determine whether such a tendency is one that ought to be allowed, promoted, or suppressed. We must first answer the distinctively moral question of whether this natural human tendency to aggression is good or valuable. When we ask, what sort of treatment do we owe each other, it is not helpful to answer by pointing out that, in virtue of our aggression, we tend to physically assault each other. The fact of this natural tendency does not generate a normative permission that endorses such actions.

John Rawls takes a distinctive approach to the use of ideas about human nature in moral and political debate. His theory of justice not only makes a place for such ideas but also serves as a model for how to generate conceptions of human nature that could serve as normatively important ideals. Rawls is concerned from the beginning with man's moral nature, not with trying to generate normative ideas from merely descriptive accounts of human tendencies to aggression, to pleasure, and the like. There are many different appropriate accounts of humans' moral nature, each account tailored to a different role. Rawls's account is a political conception, an account of our moral nature relevant to our role as citizens. His theory of justice does not rely on other accounts of human nature, although it makes room for such accounts in political decision making. Generally, his approach involves identifying a framework of value implicit in a sphere of human endeavor and then determining what the moral nature of a person must be in order for them to find value in such a sphere.

Human Nature, Politics, and Justice as Fairness

What is the place, in a just Rawlsian society, of accounts of human nature in matters of moral debate and public policy? Rawls's own justice as fairness, his theory of political justice, makes use of a "thin" account of human nature: an account of natural, human ends and capacities that are shared by or universal to all human beings insofar as they are capable of being citizens of a democratic society. A person's full set of ends will be this narrow set supplemented by individual circumstances, personal preferences, and so on. Rawls sometimes seems to hold that values found in this full set, including perfectionist values, may be used to justify the use of political power, but only when the question is not one of basic social justice. Rawls focuses on the basic structure of society as the first question of justice because the design of the basic structure has profound implications for our ability to pursue our lives in society with others. This basic structure consists of the underlying political, economic, and social institutions of society, including such things as a constitution, a system of competitive markets, and the legal structure of the family. Basic social justice involves the justice of these basic institutions. A great many significant moral and even political matters do not fall under the umbrella of basic social justice, however, such as the decision to use public funds to support a parks system in one's town, or the question of the obligations of a child to an infirm parent.

A *public reason* is the framework of reason a society uses to make collective decisions. Rawls defends the claim that individuals have a moral obligation to remain in this framework when debating matters of basic justice in certain public contexts, such as in the legislature. The content of public reason is given by the political values. These values, which constitute the set of values we have an obligation to make use of when justifying to each other our votes on matters of basic social justice, come out of an analysis of the role of citizen. This is the role that people have in a fair system of social cooperation, the political role of persons.

We lay out Rawls's analysis of this role and consider the place of nonpolitical values in a just society, particularly the place of perfectionist values that describe natural human ends. We then develop a framework for debate about fairness in sport that relies on a thin account of human nature. This framework is consistent with the requirements of justice and parallels Rawls's own account in significant ways by being an account of the role of athlete—that is, of a person's moral nature conceived as a sport participant.

Rawls endorses a version of a liberal principle of legitimacy. "Our exercise of political power is proper and hence justifiable only when it is exercised in accordance with a constitution the essentials of which all citizens may reasonably be expected to endorse in light of principles and ideals acceptable to them as reasonable and rational" (2005, p. 217). The intuitive idea is that in a liberal society the power of government—political power—is the collective power of the citizens of the society. When this coercive power is exercised, its use must be justifiable to the citizens. The use of the collective power of the citizenry must respect each citizen as reasonable and rational, and we thus need some criteria to evaluate our procedures for making use of the government's coercive power. Rawls answers this problem with his liberal principle of legitimacy. The constitution spells out fair terms of cooperation that are acceptable to citizens as reasonable and rational, and it specifies the institutions of society that make up its basic structure, within which we each pursue our lives, and that are the embodiment of these terms. So the exercise of political power is legitimate when it is used in accord with a just constitution.

The liberal principle of legitimacy implies what Rawls calls a duty of civility. This is a moral, not a legal, duty. Citizens must "be able to explain to one another on those fundamental questions [of basic social justice] how the principles and policies they advocate and vote for can be supported by the political values of public reason. This duty also involves a willingness to listen to others and a fair-mindedness in deciding when accommodations to their views should reasonably be made" (2005, p. 217). The idea here is that if we need to exercise our political power "in accordance with a constitution the essentials of which all citizens may reasonably be expected to endorse," then when we are engaged in evaluating that constitution itself, along with other matters of basic social justice, we must conduct our evaluation in terms that are acceptable to citizens *as reasonable and rational* and not on the basis of values found only in particular *conceptions of the good*. It is for this reason that one might think that Rawls rejects appeals to particular views of human nature in moral and political debate, including debates about fairness in sport. The political values we are to stick to when evaluating the basic structure are of two kinds. The first comes out of the theory of justice and its two principles, and includes the basic rights and so on. The second kind of political values includes the values of public reason. These govern our exercise of reason and require that debate be "free and public as well as informed and reasonable" (Rawls, 2001, p. 91) and so restrict us to using public rules of inference and judgment.

When we are evaluating the basic structure of society, justice requires that all reasonable persons limit the premises in their arguments to content that is acceptable to all as reasonable persons, regardless of their full comprehensive conception of the good, be they Catholics or Kantians. This restricted content includes especially what Rawls refers to as the two model conceptions of democratic society understood as a fair system of social cooperation and of persons considered as free and equal, reasonable and rational citizens of such a society. Further, justice requires that we all accept the duty of civility. This means we agree to limit ourselves to using just these political values when evaluating the basic structure. Public reason consists of these substantive values as well as the formal requirements on our methods of reasoning and rules of evidence and so on, within which we are morally obligated to remain when publicly justifying to each other our vote on matters of basic social justice. It is the framework within which we as a society collectively deliberate when we make collective decisions about how to use our collective—political—power.

To engage in public reason is to appeal to the principles and values of a political conception of justice. Such a conception of justice has three features.

1. It applies to the basic structure of society.
2. It can be presented independently of any comprehensive doctrine, which is a comprehensive religious, ethical, or philosophical view that "applies to all subjects and covers all values" (Rawls, 2001, p. 14)
3. It can be worked out from fundamental ideas implicit in the public political culture of a constitutional regime (Rawls, 2005, pp. 452–53).

In a society that is well ordered by a conception of justice, there is some agreement, but not universal agreement, about value and the dictates of morality. There is agreement precisely on the political conception of justice, and the citizens have a shared sense of (political) justice. The political conception of justice is a kind of module that fits into any person's reasonable comprehensive religious, philosophical, or ethical view, each with an attached system of final ends—that is, a conception of the good. Each distinct, reasonable, comprehensive doctrine will contain the elements for a deeper justification of the political conception of justice.

There are two contrasts to appreciate here: that between a public and a nonpublic reason and that between a comprehensive and a noncomprehensive doctrine. A public reason derives its content from a specific kind of noncomprehensive doctrine, a political conception of justice. A nonpublic reason gets its content from some comprehensive or partially comprehensive doctrine. What makes a doctrine comprehensive or partially comprehensive is just that it refers to values that cannot be worked out from ideas implicit in the public political culture of a liberal society. Thus, a comprehensive or partially comprehensive doctrine does something other than give an account of the *role of citizen*. Examples of nonpublic reasons are those of any voluntary association, such as a church, club, or scientific or sporting association. Each of these will have standards of reasoning and values that do not fall out of the idea of society as a system of fair cooperation among free and equal citizens.

Rawls does not hold that we are morally bound by the constraints of public reason in all circumstances. There are three kinds of cases where we may permissibly cite nonpolitical values. First, Rawls holds that public reason binds us when we are in certain kinds of public settings, such as in a legislature, and we justify our positions on matters of basic social justice. However, he amends this claim with a proviso. Nonpolitical values taken from a comprehensive doctrine, including references to human nature, may be used at any time, provided that "in due course public reasons, given by a reasonable political conception, are presented sufficient to support whatever the comprehensive doctrines are introduced to support" (2005, pp. xlix–l). Rawls recognizes that referring to values that are nonpolitical may be necessary to make it prudentially feasible to pass even legislation that is required as a matter of basic justice. Citing one's own comprehensive doctrine in this kind of case serves the purpose of publicly demonstrating one's own commitment to the political values from within one's most deeply held commitments; it demonstrates that one's endorsement of the political value of, for example, equal liberty is genuine. In addition, the proviso allows one to cite religious values in pursuit of a goal clearly required by the two principles—such as when Martin Luther King Jr. cited biblical texts when calling for the elimination of formal, institutionalized inequality in treatment on the basis of race. It may even be that the citing of religious values is at times necessary to motivate progress toward justice.

The second case is the case of nonpublic reasons. A church has a different reason—a framework of judgment and inference—than a scientific association does, and both of these reasons are nonpublic reasons. Rawls says, "These associations have diverse aims and purposes, and within the limits of political justice, they quite rightly view themselves in their own way" (2001, p. 92). So a private, voluntary association will have its own nonpublic reason based on its particular aims and purposes. Rawls does not think that the political and private spheres are completely separate and disconnected, each governed in entirety by its own set of principles. Rather, private associations are indirectly bound by the principles of political justice. These principles are not meant to regulate voluntary associations internally; for example, Rawls's difference principle, which says that societal institutions must be set up to maximize the share of social resources of the least advantaged social position, seems ill suited to the task of regulating the sharing of income within a family.[1] But from the point of view of justice, we are equal citizens first, and political justice holds "in and through" all nonpolitical or private associations (Rawls, 2001, p. 166). Political justice sets boundaries on what is permissible within a private, voluntary association. Excommunication is not enforced through our common coercive power. Each church is entitled to establish its own grounds for membership. However, a right of apostasy is guaranteed. Your right to leave your church is enforced by the state, and the church may not stop you from leaving. A parent's injunction to a child to clean his room is not a state matter, but access to education is.

The final case is that of legitimacy. The idea here is that a legislature may legitimately apportion money to an area of human pursuit in a way not required by justice if this apportionment is the outcome of a legitimate political process and does not implicate the justice of the basic structure. Indeed, it may be legitimate even if it violates, strictly speaking, the principles of justice. The question that arises in these sorts of cases is on what terms the debate should proceed when the issue is not one of basic social justice. Rawls sometimes seems to hold that the limits of public reason do not fully apply even in all political contexts. "My aim is to consider first the strongest case where the political questions concern the most fundamental matters. If we need not honor the limits of public reason here, it would seem we need not honor them anywhere. Should they hold here, we can then proceed to other cases. Still, I grant that it is usually highly desirable to settle political questions by invoking the political values of public reason. Yet this may not always be so" (Rawls, 2005, p. 215).

If we stick to the constraints of public reason with regard to matters of basic justice and establish background justice, then the problem that public reason is introduced to solve becomes much less acute. "The main point is that there should be a good faith commitment not to appeal to [perfectionist values] to settle the constitutional essentials and basic matters of justice. Fundamental justice must be achieved first. After that a democratic electorate may devote large resources to grand projects in art and science if it so chooses" (Rawls, 2001, p. 152). Once a just basic structure is in place, each citizen is guaranteed the fair value of their political liberties by the first principle of justice, and so each person has substantively, not merely formally, equal political power. At least, each has equal say in how our common coercive authority is used.

Beyond Basic Social Justice

Sticking to the limits of public reason, so important when considering the choice of principles of justice and their application to the basic structure, is less important once such a structure is implemented and secure and we are no longer talking about it. Most acts of a legislature do not implicate the basic structure. Perhaps we need not restrict ourselves to the political values alone when debating matters other than those of basic justice because the conditions for the legitimate exercise of political power are already in place. The outcome determined by a democratic electorate, whatever it is, is legitimate under these conditions—unless it undermines the very conditions that allow for the legitimate exercise of political power in the first place. This outcome can be legitimate even if the outcome of the legislature conflicts with the substantive requirements of justice.

There will inevitably be cases of political matters that cannot be decided on the basis of political values alone, such as the apportionment of public monies for projects in the arts or for funding a national Olympic committee. In such cases, to reach a decision, we must bring other values to bear on the issue. The question we face is how to extend the account of public reason in a way that remains true to the liberal principle of legitimacy and the duty of civility in marking the line between values we might permissibly cite and those we might still have a moral duty to avoid. We can look to Rawls's own procedure for guidance here. Rawls proceeds by looking for ideas and values implicit in liberal society. We would seek ideas and values implicit in a given practice or procedure to generate an appropriate model conception of the person to give us a substantive, though still appropriately thin, account of human nature. The sense of "thin" meant here is that the account of human nature is not comprehensive but is tied to a particular role of persons. For example, with respect to sporting associations, we look to give an account of the role of sport participant.

Rawls himself makes use of an account of human nature. In order to generate his account of public reason, he begins with two model conceptions, of society and of the person, that he finds implicit in liberal democratic culture. Society is conceived of as a fair system of cooperation between citizens conceived of as free and equal, from one generation to the next. The idea is that a liberal democratic society is a fair system of cooperation. A system of social cooperation is not simply a system of coordinated social activity. In a centrally planned society, with each individual's set of duties and benefits simply assigned by the central planner, social activity is coordinated, but this is not a system where individuals are cooperating. Cooperation, says Rawls, "is guided by publicly recognized rules and procedures that those cooperating accept and regard as properly regulating their conduct" (2005, p. 16). The idea of cooperation implies the idea of fair terms of cooperation. These terms must be publicly recognized and acceptable to the participants as reasonable.

The model conception of the person as citizen involves two moral powers. The first is the capacity for a sense of justice, which is "the capacity to understand, to apply, and to act from (not merely in accordance with) the principles of political justice that specify the fair terms of social cooperation" (Rawls, 2001, pp. 18–19). We must be able to act *from* the principles that specify fair terms of cooperation, not merely in accordance with them, because what we are engaged in is cooperation and not simply a system of coordinated activity. A society could perhaps train its citizens to act in accordance with Rawls's principles of justice using classical conditioning and a complex system of stimuli. But this society would fail to be a system of cooperation among free citizens. Rawls conceives the idea that society is a system of cooperation to be implicit in the liberal democratic tradition. That we ought to act from, and not merely in accord with, principles of justice is a development of this idea, not an argument for it.

The second moral power is the capacity for a conception of the good. Rawls describes this as "the capacity to have, to revise, and rationally to pursue a conception of the good. Such a conception is an ordered family of final ends and aims which specifies a person's conception of what is of value in human life, or, alternatively, of what is regarded as a fully worthwhile life" (Rawls and Kelly, 2001, p. 19). Our capacity for a conception of the good is our capacity to value and to assign our lives a purpose or structure in accord with our system of values. Citizens have not only this capacity but also a more or less determinate conception of the good. That is, all citizens maintain an actual system of final ends that they act in society to advance. This idea of a determinate conception of the good should be broadly understood; it includes such values as our relationships with our families and institutions that we respect and want to flourish. When we have these kinds of attachments, we view our own flourishing as involving the flourishing of others. The idea of rational advantage given by a conception of the good, then, is not assumed to be merely self-interested.

This model conception of the person is directly implied by the model conception of society. The two moral powers are required in order for a citizen to be a participant in a fair system of cooperation. Without the first moral power, a capacity for a sense of justice, social cooperation would be impossible. This is especially pertinent in the face of reasonable pluralism of conceptions of the good. Rawls takes this pluralism to be an unavoidable and persistent fact of human existence. Without this reasonable pluralism, together with the fact of a moderate scarcity of resources, "there would be no occasion for the virtue of justice" (Rawls, 1999, p. 110). The fact that people pursue varied ends and make conflicting claims on available resources requires us to come to fair terms when deciding how to share these limited resources. Given these conditions of reasonable pluralism and moderate scarcity, citizens must possess a capacity for a sense of justice in order to cooperatively participate in a fair system that determines the division of social advantages.

Citizens must have a capacity for a conception of the good because without it there is no point to cooperation. This does not imply, though, that we are *only* motivated by our conception of the good. Rawls's picture of moral psychology is not Hobbes's, in which the reasonable is reduced to the rational. If we had no ends, then there would be nothing to pursue, and the problem of reasonable pluralism would never arise. There would be no occasion for justice. This is also why we must conceive of citizens as having a concrete conception of the good, in addition to the bare capacity. It is our determinate conception that guides us in our estimation of the value of social advantages. Our conceptions of the good give each of us our motivation for participating in a cooperative system for mutual advantage—emphasis here on the *mutual*; it is, after all, a *fair* system of cooperation.

So in order to be capable of being participants in a fair system of cooperation, citizens must have both a capacity for a sense of fairness and a concrete set of values. But the commitment to fairness is in no way reducible to a concern for the good. This is distinctive of Rawls's approach to the question of justice, in contrast to what he calls a teleological approach. A teleological moral theory begins with an account of the good, often a single good—pleasure, for example, in utilitarianism— and then defines justice in terms of that pre-moral good. Central to the idea of a teleological theory is that judgments about the good can be made independently of any considerations of right or fairness. Rawls embraces a deontological approach, where the good cannot be fully specified independently of justice.

In *Political Liberalism,* the deontological quality of Rawls's thought can be expressed by the phrase "the reasonable constrains the rational." Persons are reasonable in virtue of having a capacity for a sense of justice and rational in virtue of having a capacity for a conception of the good (and a determinate conception of the good). The distinction between the two is meant to be an intuitive one. The boss's son who refuses to do his part on a project while being insulated from any threat of losing his job is said to be unreasonable, but not necessarily irrational. Without a conflict between what is rational for different people, there is no need for the virtue of justice at all. But when the two conflict, justice constrains the rational. Those who refuse to restrict their pursuit of their conception of the good by considerations of fairness are said to be unreasonable. This is one sense of what it is for us to be reasonable: we are willing to constrain what we count as good by considerations of justice. Still, the rational is independent, in the sense that our principles of justice do not fully determine our conceptions of the good. We have two distinct moral powers, two distinct sources of motivation.

What Rawls has given us in his model conception of the citizen is a thin account of human nature appropriate to the role of citizen. Persons conceived as citizens have as their nature two moral powers. From this account we also get an account of human ends. Whatever other ends we might have, we have as two of our higher-order interests the development and exercise of the two moral powers. It is on this basis that Rawls argues for his principles of justice. They will allow and promote the development and exercise of the two moral powers. We get substantive limits on what pursuits will be permissible in society, but within these limits the individual's freedom to follow her desired ends—her conception of the good—is secured. Whatever one's conception of the good is, so long as it approaches being a reasonable conception, the development of the two moral powers is necessary to pursue this conception cooperatively in a society, and thus the development and exercise of these two moral powers will be of tremendous importance. The development of the two powers will have special value from *within* each of the many reasonable conceptions of the good held by the citizens of a just liberal society.

Human Nature and Sports

We have already established that an account of human nature may permissibly be cited in arguments regarding sport in multiple spheres, from the legislature to the internal deliberations of a sport association. Rawls also provides a model of how to generate an account of human nature for purposes of achieving reflective equilibrium in the realm of sport, by giving an account of the values implicit in sport and an account of the role of sport participant. We should not simply survey existing attitudes about sport and somehow aggregate the preferences expressed, but rather we must look to the practice itself. This is not just a survey of preferences; the reasonable is doing real work here. Such an account of sport can help us decide where to apportion money for, say, sports programs in public schools or funding for Olympic athletes. These kinds of funding are probably not required in any sort of direct way by the two principles of justice. We have a duty to ensure that a wide variety of practices and pursuits flourish in our society in order to encourage the development and exercise of the two moral powers of the citizens. But we have no duty to promote any one specific pursuit. Which practices in particular receive the active assistance of the society as a whole through the use of the collective political power of the citizens is a matter left up to the democratic electorate.

Given the widespread appeal of sport, and its appeal from within a diverse array of comprehensive doctrines, it seems that some such funding and assistance is likely. The market may fail to provide sufficient access to amateur leagues and so on. Though professionals can function in the market as entertainers, this is not so for the vast majority of amateur leagues. Giving an account of the role of sport participant can help us decide what to fund and what conditions to attach to the funding and other societal advantages that might be conferred on any particular sport or sporting association.[2] This account can also guide us in developing rules to govern sport from within private sport associations—including rules about the use of performance-enhancing drugs and other technologies.

We now take up two broad questions about drugs and sport in relation to Rawls's account of justice and politics. First, what room is there for a rich conception of sport in Rawls's account? Second, how might conduct within sport be regulated, consistent with Rawls's account of justice and liberties?

Sport in a Just Society

Consider more carefully Rawls's description of the second of the two moral powers: "The capacity for a conception of the good is the capacity to form, to revise, and rationally to pursue a conception of one's rational advantage or good" (1999, p. 19). He adds that in addition to these moral powers,

> persons also have at any given time a determinate conception of the good that they try to achieve. Such a conception must not be understood narrowly but rather as including a conception of what is valuable in human life. Thus, a conception of the good normally consists of a more or less determinate scheme of final ends, that is, ends we want to realize for their own sake, as well as attachments to other persons and loyalties to various groups and associations. These attachments and loyalties give rise to devotions and affections, and so the flourishing of the persons and associations who are the objects of these sentiments is also part of our conception of the good. We also connect with such a conception a view of our relation to the world—religious, philosophical, and moral—by reference to which the value and significance of our ends and attachments are understood. (pp. 19–20)

Some determinate conception of the good and the ends appropriate to it, the quest for flourishing, the significance of attachments to persons and associations, and the importance of our relation to the world, these central concepts in Rawls's account provide ample room for a rich and thick conception of the role of sport in human life and society. The concepts may not necessarily apply for all persons; people may have quite different conceptions of what constitutes flourishing and how to reach it. But for countless people around the globe, judging by the multitudes that participate in sport, follow sport, or watch the Olympic games, sport can play an important role in an overall "conception of what is valuable in human life." Later we will return to what may account for the importance of sport across a vast multitude of cultures and times; for now it is sufficient to establish that there is ample room for sport in a Rawlsian worldview and that to the extent sport becomes part of persons' determinate conception of the good, a component of their flourishing, it is a manifestation of one of the two moral powers persons must have. Sport, therefore, may be not merely permissible in a Rawlsian world; it can be one reasonable way of fulfilling something that is required, a particular conception of the good, of ends, of what is to be valued.

Rawls and Rules

We now turn to the question of how sport can be regulated in a way consistent with Rawls's account of justice and liberties. Set aside rules that have as their primary justification "because I say so!" and we are left with rules that are justified as the outcome of a mutually agreed process and by their organic relationship with the activity in question. Rules evolve as practices and practitioners change. Good rules in sport evolve in relationship to an underlying conception of meaning in the sport, which is itself understood in relation to a conception of human flourishing, a partially comprehensive view of the good, and, we argue later, a thin but nevertheless important account of human nature.

Rules, of course, are a general feature of competitions, as limiting cases illuminate. Lee Atwater, the bare-knuckled political consultant, was reputed to have said of a losing candidate that he forgot that the rules of politics are the same as the rules of knife fighting: there are no rules. Then there is Calvinball, in which the only rule is that you cannot have the same rule twice. Not all activities governed by formal rules are sports, however; take chess, crossword-puzzle tournaments, pie baking, and, possibly, the various "reality" contests that infest contemporary American television. These contests generally lack the physical dimensions—strength, speed, grace, or stamina—that in various combinations appear to characterize sport.

And not all physical activities, even those that require considerable athleticism, are sports. Professional wrestling is physically demanding, calling on strength and technique. But it is a scripted morality play, not a contest; the outcome is preordained. Ballet is another example.

Authentic contests, including sporting events, appear to share certain features. Vicious externalities, such as bribes to officials supervising the contest, are prohibited, as are efforts to sabotage competitors' equipment, food, or drink. Physically disabling one's competition—as the figure skater Tanya Harding arranged to be done to Nancy Kerrigan—so clearly violates the meaning of sport that whether figure skating had a rule that expressly forbade it is irrelevant. Conspiring to assault a person is a crime and is also unethical. But suppose Harding found some noncriminal way to ensure that Kerrigan was unable to compete against her—say, intentionally giving Kerrigan bad directions to the arena. Even if no specific skating rule was broken, that action would result at best in a hollow, meaningless victory, one achieved not by athletic talent honed to perfection but by cunning and ruthlessness that had nothing to do with performance in the rink.

Sport is certainly a rule-governed activity, but the Harding-Kerrigan case suggests that the rules for a sport do not so much constitute its meaning as manifest imperfectly and incompletely a meaning that is constructed in some other manner. Rules for sport and other competitions do many things. One crucial function of rules is to determine what differences among competitors are permitted to make a difference in the outcome and what differences among competitors are not. In pie baking, for example, every competitor should have an equal chance to use a suitable oven, one that bakes evenly and at a predictable temperature. It would be unfair to give one baker a precisely regulated oven and force other competitors to use broken-down, unreliable ovens. Whatever factors should decide the winning pie baker, the quality of the oven is not one.

One dubious view holds that rules constitute the sport and stipulate its meaning, more or less without remainder. But, of course, the rules of sports can change. A brief reflection suggests that such changes are far from arbitrary. Baseball has been striking in the durability of its basic rules, giving support to Rawls's assertion that it is the best of all games. But even baseball has adjusted as the game has evolved. The pitchers mound was lowered to reconfigure the balance between pitcher and hitter; a lower mound favors the batter, resulting in more hits and more runs.

Basketball has had more frequent and dramatic rules changes. When very tall and athletic players arrived capable of reaching above the basket to knock shots away, goal-tending was defined and banned. As physically imposing players began to dominate by establishing themselves close to the basket, the three-second lane was created to keep offensive players from camping under the hoop, and a three-point line was drawn to reward long-range shooting and to force defenses to guard the perimeter, which also opened up interior passing and slashing drives to the rim. Speed, grace, passing, and shooting were being eclipsed by sheer size and strength; rules changes restored their place in the game.

There are two distinct goals one might have internal to participation in a sport. The first is to play the game fairly and well under a fair set of rules. The second is to win. Sometimes, these goals come into conflict. There are multiple ways to solve this conflict of desires. Some might say we are unreasonable to hold on to the desire to win in this situation. Others might say we are irrational to hold to fairness. But our conclusion is neither of these. Rather, we say that we want to win, but not unfairly. My desire to win is not a desire to win by any means necessary. Sometimes my desire to win will go unrealized. But, there is nothing irrational, unreasonable, or psychologically implausible about that.[3]

Many factors undoubtedly contributed to the evolution of the rules of basketball, among them the commercial interests of professional team owners, broadcast networks, players, and advertising sponsors. The issue is not whether such interests had any influence; surely they did, but these entities were also subject to the shared understandings among all those who love basketball as to what made the game worth playing and watching. Such shared understandings for well-established sports exist; they shape the evolution of each sport, including its rules. A vital component of these shared understandings is a sense of what differences among competitors should and should not affect the outcomes, and for sport in general, and for each particular sport, the primary differences affecting outcome should be some combination of natural talents and the manner in which those talents are brought to their current state. In short, sports exalt natural talents and their virtuous perfection, and every sport calls forth its own mix of particular talents. Sprinting honors acceleration and speed; weightlifting emphasizes explosive strength and technique. Other sports, the decathlon for example, require wide arrays of talents. Team sports such as baseball, basketball, and soccer can benefit from different combinations of talents at different roles or positions. All such sports require persistence, hard work, intense concentration, and discipline.

Given these connections, it is unsurprising that sports organizations subscribe to and enforce a set of rules that incorporate a particular understanding of talents as "natural" and that prohibit certain means of augmenting or enhancing those talents. There are tricky cases, like hypoxic chambers, that are not easily resolved, but to have a minimally coherent account of sport, we must have some account of human nature in sport. From that account flows a set of guidelines about the kind of arguments that need to be made, even if the account does not easily or directly settle all questions for us. But why should we expect it to? Judgment is an undeniable part of life.

Sports and the Just Society

Can John Rawls, unsurpassed philosopher of justice and lover of baseball, help us understand the place of sport and of the concept of "natural talents" in a society that seeks to establish justice through fundamental political, social, and economic institutions and basic liberties? We believe that giving sports organizations this social role is consistent with a Rawlsian conception of a just society. Persons necessarily possess the moral power to have a conception of what is valuable in human life and the capacity to connect that conception of what is good and valuable with "a view of our relation to the world." As embodied creatures, rather than vaporous clouds of consciousness, the relation of that consciousness and our capacity for intentional action to our biological bodies is an unavoidable component of our relation to the world. To put it bluntly, any conception of what is *humanly* good and valuable must address the reality that, as humans, we each have a body, and it must provide for us guidance as to how our body is to regarded and treated.

Our bodies are our all-purpose means for pursuing any ends in the world at all. They are the manifestation of self in space and time. They are malleable to some degree, which can cause us to differ in our judgments whether altering the internal state of the body is permissible, through either external technology or more direct means.

Some "comprehensive doctrines" regard the body as a nuisance and distraction, counseling indifference to our appetites and desires, or even mortification of the flesh. Other doctrines emphasize the body as the locus of sensations and commend surrender to the pleasures of the flesh. Whether any of these would pass the Rawlsian test of reasonableness is not at issue here; we need only show that reasonably comprehensive doctrines can include the view that the intentional perfection of physical excellences, through sport or similar activities, is something to be valued and a component of human flourishing.

The near-universal practice of sport, formal or informal, across times and cultures is one important piece of evidence. Global interest in the Olympic games is another. Sport in this sense is a practice that celebrates physical excellence perfected by intentional activity. It connects our capacity for moral agency with our biological embodiment in a direct and immediate way. Discipline and dedication, finely honed and exhaustively practiced technique, and the willingness to suffer are merely a few of the virtues that transform raw natural talent into polished athletic performance. Frankly, we are unable to think of a virtue important to achieving excellence in sport that is not also valuable to the flourishing of individuals and communities in many other realms of life.

Some critics assert that a fundamental aspect of being human is our relationship to technology. They point to technologies from composite vaulting poles to resilient synthetic running tracks as evidence that performance-enhancing technologies are already ubiquitous in sport. They argue further that drugs like anabolic steroids, biologicals like synthetic EPO, and genetic manipulation should be regarded merely as additional technologies, no different in their significance or moral acceptability from modern poles or tracks.

Critics have full liberty to advance such arguments and, indeed, to set up their own sport associations that embrace any or all of these technologies (unless through fair processes and legitimate public reasoning, particular uses are prohibited—out of concern for public health, for example). The sport of power lifting, not to be confused with weight lifting, has taken this route, with multiple associations springing into existence with extremely wide variations in their tolerance toward performance-enhancing drugs. (We leave aside for now the problem of a voluntary sport association promoting or prominently turning a blind eye toward behaviors associated with criminal activity, such as the sale of prohibited substances.)

What matters here is that a thin conception of human nature underlying sport that distinguishes between acceptable uses of technology, such as those that require the athlete's active engagement and mastery, and unacceptable uses of technology, such as those that confer significant competitive advantage by directly and radically altering the body's chemistry or genetics, is reasonable in Rawls's sense. That is, although this view may be shaped by content-rich conceptions of the good and of what is humanly valuable, a view that embraces drug-free sport can satisfy the basic principles of justice. Furthermore, to the extent that sport takes place within voluntary associations, it has considerable latitude in determining its own practices and rules, subject to the constraints of basic fairness.

Critics of antidoping in sport will find in Rawls ample support for their liberty to advance whatever public reasons they wish to change the rules of sport. They will also find support for their right to challenge whatever understandings of our relation to our bodies, and of human nature and the natural, they believe under-pin current antidoping policies; these conceptions of the good, which may include what are sometimes called perfectionist values, are fair game as well. But Rawls also supports those of us who believe that antidoping is important in sport for prudential, public health reasons (which are, in Rawls's terms, public reasons) or for reasons based on a conception of what is good and valuable in human life.

Unearned Gifts

One confusion remains to be dealt with: the claim that because natural talents are "unearned," justice requires a redress, perhaps in the form of some sort of talent handicapping or talent equalizing. Critics of Rawls point out that justice as fairness explicitly rejects the idea "that income and wealth, and the good things in life generally, should be distributed according to moral worth" (1999, p. 310). Our talents, even our character, are not things we "deserve." "It seems to be one of the fixed points of our considered judgments that no one deserves his place in the distribution of native endowments, any more than one deserves one's initial starting place in society. The assertion that a man deserves the superior character that enables him to make the effort to cultivate his abilities is equally problematic; for his character depends in large part on fortunate family and social circumstances for which he can claim no credit" (1999, p. 104).

So, if we do not deserve morally either our natural talents (which are, after all, the product of a "natural lottery") or our ability to virtuously perfect those talents, how would a just society deal with such differences? Rawls offers an illuminating distinction in the form of a sports analogy: "After a game one often says that the losing side deserved to win. Here one does not mean that the victors are not entitled to claim the championship, or whatever spoils go to the winner. One means instead that the losing team displayed to a higher degree the skills and qualities that the game calls forth, and the exercise of which gives the sport its appeal. Therefore the losers truly deserved to win but lost out as a result of bad luck, or from other contingencies that caused the contest to miscarry" (1999, p. 314).

The distinction here is between *entitlement* and *moral worth*. Justice as fairness is concerned with establishing a set of fundamental political, social, and economic institutions. Those institutions set rules for distributing shares of social resources. If one abides by those rules, one is entitled to the shares of resources one legitimately acquires. A larger share of resources is not evidence of superior moral worth; nor does moral worth in itself entitle one to a larger share of resources. There is ample room in justice as fairness for those who are willing to work harder and longer, as well as for those who have special talents, to be entitled to larger shares, as long as the basic institutions satisfy the difference principle that requires the structure of the overall scheme to be to the advantage of the least advantaged positions in society. Justice as fairness does not require equal shares for all; it does require equal rights for all and equal opportunity for all. In particular, social advantages—class, wealth, connections—should not be readily convertible into unequal shares of social resources. Natural talents, on the other hand, may entitle one to larger shares of social resources as long as the difference principle, which focuses on representative positions within society over a lifetime and not on distributions to particular individuals, is satisfied. A society that fails to value hard work or talents may result in a more equal distribution of resources, but it may also make the least advantaged worse off than they might be in a society that was mindful of justice but also rewarded work and talent.

Rawls raises the principle of redress and its relationship to desert: "This is the principle that undeserved inequalities call for redress; and because inequalities of birth and natural endowment are undeserved, these inequalities are to be somehow compensated for" (1999, p. 86). But "the difference principle is not of course the principle of redress. It does not require society to try to even out handicaps as if all were expected to compete on a fair basis in the same race" (p. 86). The difference principle, he explains, achieves some of the aim of the principle of redress, not by handicapping the talented but by transforming

> the aims of the basic structure so that the total scheme of institutions no longer emphasizes social efficiency and technocratic value. The difference principle represents, in effect, an agreement to regard the distribution of natural talents as a common asset and to share in the greater social and economic benefits made possible by the complementarities of this distribution. Those who have been favored by nature, whoever they are, may gain from their good fortune only on terms that improve the situation of those who have lost out. . . . No one deserves his greater natural capacity nor merits a more favorable starting place in society. But, of course, this is no reason to ignore, much less to eliminate these distinctions. Instead, the basic structure can be arranged so that these contingencies work for the good of the least fortunate. (p. 87)

Some interpreters of Rawls have taken this line to mean that we are to regard each person's talents as a common asset, which would violate the individual integrity of the person. But as the passage indicates, it is not *my* talents that are a common asset but the distribution of talents in society, and "the basic structure can be arranged so that these contingencies work for the good of the least fortunate," while at the same time those who work harder and longer earn more. My living is made off of my talents, used how I wish them to be used. We are to set up the basic structure so that people using their individual talents to make their own living benefits everyone. Rawls talks about this as a "division of labor" between society and the individual. "If this division of labor can be established, individuals and associations are then left free to advance their own ends more effectively within the framework of the basic structure, secure in the knowledge that elsewhere in the social system the necessary corrections to preserve background justice are being made" (2005, p. 269). Individuals are responsible for advancing their own ends even as the basic structure is responsible for guaranteeing a background of fairness within which these ends are pursued.

We find it interesting, but perhaps not surprising, that John Rawls, skilled player and lover of baseball, reached for sport metaphors to illuminate important aspects of *A Theory of Justice*. Society is not required to handicap talents so that all competitors in a race have equal chances at winning. A team can deserve to win without being entitled to the spoils of victory. There is no intrinsic injustice if victory goes to the talented and dedicated. Injustice arises when differences in the natural or social lottery bias the fundamental political, social, and economic institutions of a society. If basic liberties are protected, fair equality of opportunity flourishes, and the institutions of the society create and distribute social resources so as to advantage those in the least advantaged social positions, then justice as fairness is being achieved. That talent and effort are recognized and rewarded with shares of social resources is not, in itself, a violation of justice as fairness. Casey Stengel was right: baseball is a game of skill. Don't be surprised if talent leads to success and its absence to failure. Or you could always become a manager.

NOTES

1. There are two principles, lexically ordered such that in evaluating candidate sets of institutions the first principle must be satisfied before the second is applied. First, each person has the same indefeasible claim to a fully adequate scheme of basic liberties, which scheme is compatible with same scheme of liberties for all. Second, social and economic inequalities are to satisfy two conditions: they are to be attached to offices and positions open to all under conditions of fair equality of opportunity, and they are to be to the greatest benefit of the least advantaged members of society (Rawls, 2001, pp. 42–43).

2. This brings to mind the case of the monopoly power granted to baseball team owners, a benefit that seems indefensible from just about any point of view except that of the owners themselves.

3. Thank you to Jon Mandle for this point.

REFERENCES

Rawls, J. 1999. *A Theory of Justice,* rev. ed. Cambridge, Mass.: Belknap Press of Harvard University Press.

———. 2005. *Political Liberalism,* expanded ed. New York: Columbia University Press.

Rawls, J., and E. Kelly. 2001. *Justice as Fairness: A Restatement.* Cambridge, Mass.: Belknap Press of Harvard University Press.

Index

Aaron, Hank, 130
Adorno, Theodor, *Aesthetic Theory*, 12–14
Agar, Nicholas, 60
agency of athletes, 132, 136–37
agrarian ideal, 121
agricultural biotechnology, x–xi
agriculture, industrial model of, 121–23
altitude training, 159, 162, 164
amniocentesis, 111
amour propre, 36
analytic truths, 89
antecedent interests, 160–62
anthropocentrism, 11–12, 95–96
antidoping, critics of, 195–96
antifoundationalist theories, 2
appeals to nature: aesthetic rationale for,
   12–14; in bioethics, 126–27; biotechnology
   and, 141–44; as both vital and problematic,
   176–78; breast-feeding and, 101–3; Buchanan
   and, 103–4; comparative examination of,
   xii–xiv; constraint-based account of, 144–46;
   definition of, ix; disability and, 55; discrimination and injustice in, 108–9; environment
   and, xi; genetic manipulation of offspring
   and, 106–8; grateful contentment and,
   110–11; history of, 98; human bodies and,
   ix–x; humility and, 114–15; as implicit, 10–12;
   Mill and, 99–100; moral rules and, 126–27;
   other species and, x–xi; policy and, xi; President's Council on Bioethics and, 104–6, 108;
   Sandel and, 100–101
Aristotle: essentialist view and, 50; Kass on, 58;
   natural philosophy of, 19–20, 38–39; point
   of equipoise and, 177; view of procreation
   of, 105
Arnhart, Larry, 51–52

artifacts: definition of, 72; ecological restoration and, 72–78; Kant and, 4–5; public policy
   and, 81–82
artificial, dualism in conceptions of, 93
athletic achievement: authenticity of, 132–33,
   136–37, 192; biotechnology for enhancement
   of, 131, 132–38; collective pride in, 130–31;
   estrangement of athletes from fans, 139–40;
   repudiation of bodies of athletes, 138–39;
   thresholds for defining, 142–43. *See also*
   sports
Atwater, Lee, 191
audience, and elite sports, 149–50

baseball: home run records in, 130, 140–41;
   performance enhancement and, 146–47;
   Rawls on, 179; rule changes in, 140–41, 192
basketball, rule changes in, 192–93
Benjamin, Walter, 13
Berry, Wendell, 121–25, 126–28
Beyond Therapy (President's Council on
   Bioethics), 58, 135–41
bioethics, appeals to nature in, 126–27. *See also*
   President's Council on Bioethics
biological versus nonbiological products, 91–92
biotechnology: agricultural, x–xi; appeals
   to nature and, 141–44; for enhancement of
   athletic performance, 131, 132–38; lack of
   transparency and, 142; pace of innovation in,
   142; President's Council on Bioethics and, ix,
   135–41; resistance to forms of, 14. *See also* enhancement technologies; genetic modification
bodies, human: appeals to nature and, ix–x; of
   athletes, repudiation of, 138–39; environmental interventions on, 64–65; genetic interventions into, 64; purpose of, 194

Émile (Rousseau), 36, 38, 40
Endangered Species Act, xi
end-of-life issues, 127–28
The End of Nature (McKibben), 85, 86, 87,
    88–89
enhancement in sports: Kass and, 57–59;
    limited approach to, 65–66; objections to, 54.
    See also performance enhancement
enhancement technologies: capacity for
    sympathy and, 61; Fukuyama and, 59–60;
    Habermas and, 62–65; justification for,
    174–75; Murray and, 65–66; opposition to,
    60–61; Sandel and, 61–62, 63–65. *See also*
    therapy/enhancement distinction
Enough (McKibben), ix, 150–51
environmental interventions on human bodies,
    64–65
environmentalism: defense of living nature,
    collective action for, 25–26; end of nature
    and, 85–86; focus of, 84; human actions and,
    88, 89–90; intrinsic goodness of nature and,
    21–22; species loss and, xi
environmental philosophy, 84–85, 86, 95–96
environmental policy and idea of nature, 71
erythropoietin (EPO): ban on, 160, 163–64;
    interest in identifying and, 162–63; spectator
    interests and, 150; WADA and, 158–59
essentialist definition of nature, 6–7
essentialist view of species: Buchanan and,
    103–6, 108; evolutionary view of species
    compared to, 50–53; Fukuyama and, 60; Kass
    and, 58
estrangement: of athletes from fans, 139–40;
    from nature, 43–44
ethics: bioethics, appeals to nature in, 126–27;
    theories of, 27n5. *See also* President's Council
    on Bioethics
evolutionary view of species, 50–53, 102

Factor X, 59–60
family farming, 121–23
fans, estrangement of athletes from, 139–40
fiction, and simulation theory, 153, 154–55
FIFA World Cup soccer, 154
Filmer, Robert, 33
"first nature," 13

food, genetically modified, x, 3–4
forests, old-growth, logging of, xi
"Frankenstein science" notion, 3–4
Freitas, Robert A., Jr., 162–63
Freud, Sigmund, 9, 46
Friedman, Theodore, 139–40
Fukuyama, Francis, 59–60, 98

genetic determinism, 107
genetic engineering, developments in, and
    conventions of culture, 2–3
genetic interventions into human bodies, 64
genetic modification: as artifactual, 5; of
    character traits of offspring, 106–8; of food,
    x, 3–4; "species barrier" and, 5–6. *See also*
    biotechnology; enhancement technologies;
    therapy/enhancement distinction
genitalia, ambiguous, 54
giftedness: ethic of, 61–62, 64, 108–9, 111, 124;
    Sandel on, 100–101
gifts, unearned, talents as, 196–98
Glo-fish, x
Glover, Jonathan, 67
good: capacity for conception of, 187–88,
    190–91; human, and value of human nature,
    65–68
goodness of nature, intrinsic, and scholastics,
    21–22, 23
government policy. *See* public policy
gradualist objections to biotechnology, 133
grateful contentment, idea of, 110–11
Green, Ronald, 98

Habermas, Jürgen, 14, 62–65, 98
habits of mind and ways of being, 124–25, 127–28
Haraway, Donna, 10
Harding, Tanya, 165, 192
Harris, John, 98
health as example of embodied normative
    discourse, 168
hematocrit (HCT), 158–59, 162
history and nature, 13
Hobbes, Thomas: social contract theory of,
    31–33, 39–40, 41–46; as strong theorist, 29, 30
Hoffe, Otfried, 14
Holland, Stephen, 142–44, 145–46